HEALERS

FORAM SHAH

ISBN: 978-93-86526-57-1

First Published: October 2017

Cover Design
Dwaipayan Mani

Distributed by

shopclues.com
power-publishers.com
readwhere.com
flipkart.com
snapdeal.com
infibeam.com
amazon.com
amazon.in
ebay.in

Contents

Chapter 1

Desperate Times!

Mommy walked into a departmental store. The air from the air-conditioner hit right on her face, blowing her hair. Yup! The air was a tad bit stronger than the usual days and that would considerably be so! The fruits and vegetables were ageing and were on the verge of rotting.

They were all lying in an old, antique looking glass compartment. They were trying to catch her eyes, one jumping above another. They were all aggressively vying for a spot in her bamboo basket.

They were all crying "me me me", some were screaming "here woman here" and few others were barking, "hey woman! Look at me. Why don't you ever see me?"

And magically mommy's head turned right towards them.

"Let us out!" They all banged against the glass.

She walked up to aisle no.7 which happened to be the last-in- line, least walked down aisle. It was isolated and had a peculiar go-away aura. She passed the aisle no.1 which was packed cheerfully with purchasers. That aisle carried "The very populous", "Exotic" and "in demand", of Chippito chips, along with the old favourite cheesy potato snacks.

Second aisle was a special aisle too. Though not as popular as first aisle, the white bread and highly processed meat was beloved by bakers and makers.

Third and fourth aisle were custom made heaven for guzzlers. Processed juice cartons, flavored healthy sodas, and crates of body building protein shakes. Ironically, it was all supposed to be healthy!

Fifth and sixth aisles were for those busy-bees, who groan and grunt, if cooking is not instant. Instant pasta, instant noodles, ready to make soups, on-the-go dinner kits. Damn!!! Devil come on earth if anything takes more than 5 minutes over here.

All these aisles products were celebrated and famed. Their demand was always higher than supply. They were not left in cold or probably forgotten like the fruits and vegetables, who were dying every day to be noticed. They never had to breathe down each other's neck, while squishing themselves against the glass; standing on top of one another at awkward angles like some gymnast experts. Or never had to endure the freezing drizzles of air conditioner. In fact, it was way too cold inside to do anything, except to whimper and bawl about how cold it is inside.

Bitter Gourd sat alone in a corner, looking at the pathetic act of his glass mates trying to sell themselves. A diminishing faint Himalayan smell wafted from him. "Weak! So weak!" He muttered to himself under his breath. "They would make a worthless army in times of war."

"What did you say mate?" Lettuce asked looking over at him cautiously.

"I said you all will make a trashy army," Bitter-Gourd spat on him.

"And you sitting alone there will make a mighty one yourself, it seems!" Lettuce argued back showing his temper.

"Alone, yes, but still a mightier one than a pack of plastic surgery cartoons that you all are!"

Lettuce made a face. Bitter-Gourd smelled a whip of him. "You reek. What were you, drenched in a tub of insecticides?"

"I was brought up by a pack of weeds. Something I am not proud of." Lettuce said soberly. Everybody knew humans spayed a lot of insecticides to kill the weeds.

"Horrible! Just horrible!" Bitter Gourd smirked, eyeing a bright red strawberry, "What a shame! She had to inject herself to enhance her colour from red to blood red. Too much pressure living up to her family name of the berries, aye, it seems!"

"She didn't ask for it! You don't know humans!" lettuce exclaimed angrily.

"Well, it seems like she did it herself. Would love to bet on it!" He spat back confidently. Right now strawberry was giving all lovey-dovey eyes to banana, who happened to be another cartoon head in the glass compartment. Apparently he was all built up. Broader from top, narrower from below!

"Bet he is on steroids!" Bitter-Gourd declared out.

"What is up with you jerk? Perhaps looking for another fight?" Lettuce asked angrily.

"No just concerned. How are these people even going to nourish bodies, especially growing children? Our job is to be full of nutrients and not to be a perfect object for selfies." Bitter- Gourd argued. "Well, it's a blessing that you guys haven't yet perished."

“Nobody had a choice, mate. Anyways, you don’t know look like you know much about the real world.” Lettuce sighed, blinking back his tears. Only a few months ago, he was separated from his wife. She was sprayed with too much of insecticide. She couldn’t endure the harsh stuff and developed a chemical reaction which turned her skin orange. She was immediately discarded in the garbage bin.

Bitter Gourd could never understand their sorrows. He was totally free from insecticides. His bitter taste was insect- repellent in itself. Also, he had a blessed upbringing. Swaying in Himalayan air on Himalayan slopes, amidst a bunch of sweet smelling roses, besides a particular temple. His ancestors were prayed and sprinkled with holy water of God everyday. Not one and all were that lucky. Ah! He had a blissful life.

Though even, Lettuce didn’t quite deny that Strawberry and Banana had a terrible reputation! Like, for instance, right now, Strawberry was cheering like cheerleader for banana, who had climbed on the top of tomato, tapping his rough back on face of tomato. Poor Tomato!

Her eyes were busy fluttering, her cheeks were blushing red. Meanwhile her man stud was flexing his muscles, pressed across the glass pane. Indeed, poor Tomato!

Truth to be told, the Tomato was indeed the most abused one amidst them. He was injected with fillers against his wish. But most agonising was watching his childhood sweetheart die a brutal death in front of himself. She, Miss Tomato was run over by a truck. He was scared, seeing her getting crushed and spilling out all her internal juices. He would stay disturbingly quiet and would sometimes hysterically mutter in his sleep about swaying in fields together and eating compost from the soil.

“Keep quiet. Will you!” Lemon would often scold others from besides. Ironically, he had to be the one to speak. A bunch of rowdy, his family were. Everybody would keep a shielded distance from them. They have been the sourest family ever. Their children would ceaselessly, round the clock leak their puss. The intensity of puss would burn other’s eyes and skin.

Though humans wouldn’t tear a lemon off with their teeth like Apples and Tomatoes or probably put it in their fruit salads, it was still a fruit to the disgust of all the fruits in the glass compartment.

"One would think the lemons would teach their kid's toilet manners, but not that crooked people! They would make a circle out of their puss to scare away all from encroaching their space." Fruits would cry.

"Lemon" Grape-fruit, the social butterfly, huffed "they are so lemony!"

"It's a nightmare to be even associated with them, encroaching their space! As if!" she exclaimed dramatically, as that was the biggest lie she had ever heard.

"Thank God; it's a vegetable-fruit and not fruit-fruit. It would be such a shame otherwise." Cherries chipped in wisely.

"Thank Goodness", they all agreed.

The Fruits were pack of arrogant people. They knew they would always have an edge over vegetables. Even though one wouldn't buy fruits for eating, they would always be bought by women to be mixed in their face packs, or probably picked up by shampoo or perfume makers.

While mommy was busy deciding what to buy, she suddenly took two steps back and walked back towards aisle no. 5

She sadly gazed at the faint glass compartment from a distance. "My daughter would never eat that."

Chapter 2

Pans and Kettles!

"The cost of vegetables has raised the roof." Mother ranted. "And this girl refuses to eat at all. She didn't even glance at her soup last night? What am I supposed to do?" She sighed worriedly as she pulled off her apron, detaching it from her neck and placing it on the table.

All the vegetables gathered around in their basket. They all had a face like thunder. "Who is it going to be today? Do you have any idea?" They all whispered to each other.

"Whoever it is, I have the gunny bag ready. Just jump in it." Lemon whispered back urgently.

"This is cruel. It's getting scarier every day to escape this storm." Chubby Cauliflower cried. "She narrowly discovered my hiding spot yesterday, when she stood on a stool and searched the entire top shelve with her stretched hands." Cauliflower would now hesitate to hide again in his usual spot, a small hole in the wall, at the corner of the top shelves. Few days back, carrot and radish were kissing each other on the very same top shelf, when mommy searched and caught them. His spot was almost discovered too. Her hands had lightly brushed against his leaf, but he swiftly managed to pull it off from under her hands.

"One by one, everybody is going to die, but it is so difficult to say goodbye." Mrs Lady Finger sobbed. "My husband liked the name okra. So we named him okra!" She sniffed as she cradled her infant son in the bamboo basket. "Now he will never get to see him grow up." She wiped her tears.

"This is our job; we were born to die." Chubby Cauliflower tried to calm Mrs. Lady Finger.

It was particularly a sensitive moment for her; as her husband was cooked to death yesterday. They had made an agreement when they had entered the house that if they were eaten on separate days, they would meet inside the body. But sadly, the girl never touched her soup last night and the entire soup, which also had her husband, was drained down the basin. They somehow tried to retrieve him back by going down the basin but alas! It was too late. He had died of his burns. She had held his hands throughout the time they tried to heal him by putting turmeric and pouring cold water on him from the sink. But his burns from the flame were too intense. They, then, even gave him a proper burial by burring him in the soil of the potted plants in the Kitchen window, along with his few leftovers which were cut during the making of the soup. Everybody who knew him spoke five kind words for him.

It was also a painful process to see vegetables getting cut daily. Their juice would flow out whenever a knife pierced through them. Then they would even be fried in hot oil on burning flame. Humans thought that the stirring sounds in pan were made by the spices when mixed with oil; but it was actually vegetables screaming for mercy. They were begging not to be treated so inhumanely. They were seething with pain. They bend; lose their shapes, and their colours become dark. Horrific! Some of them even turned ashy dark on high flame due to the negligence of this barbaric people. Yesterday a bunch of Apples were skinned alive to make Apple salad. It was grotesque!

"I am a widow now!" Miss Lady Finger cried, devastated; unable to come to terms with the death of her husband. "I hope, I am chosen today and get digested quickly in the intestine. I don't want to live anymore. Please take care of my son!" She pleaded chubby Cauliflower.

"Don't say that. He is in a much better place." Chubby Cauliflower calmed her, by rubbing his hands soothingly on her arms. Others too surrounded her trying to cheer her up.

"Really?" she asked hopefully.

"Of course, Yes! He is in heaven. He did his job well on earth. He was a good man!" Miss Lady Leek spoke kindly in her British accent, as she took her hand in her hands.

Overwhelmed by listening to Miss Lady Leek, Mrs Lady Finger broke in tears.

"What about my infant son?" Mrs Lady Finger asked astounded, "He will miss his father."

"He is just an infant. He will soon forget all about him." Chubby Cauliflower balmed the disturbed Mrs Lady Finger by taking her in his arms.

Miss Lady Leek looked at them dazzled, while still stroking Lady Finger's hand. Love was a foreign concept for her. She was born in a laboratory of Britain. She was artificial as they call it! It was a successful experiment in their laboratory. The two scientists, who invented her, were so thrilled on her birth that they called her, their lady, 'lady treasure'! They smelled her and called her a key to a treasure. She had a faint odour to her just like how a real Leek would have. They loved her. First thing in the morning, they kissed her adoringly. They taught her their perfect British manners. Educated her on how to sit, walk and talk like a proper lady.

Her birth was sensational news. Everybody wanted to capture her in their cameras. One fine day, she was placed for auction in a hall. It gradually occurred to her, that the Scientists were selling her. They let all potential buyers grope and violate her. They touched and smelled her indecently. In a flash, her trust was broken like a shattered mirror and slowly her love faded away. By the fall of the hammer, she was sold to a high-profile beautician that evening. The beautician desired to use her in face packs; so she could tell the world her experience of using an artificial leek on her face via her blog. She was placed high on the shelf of the refrigerator and after few days, was joined by another elderly fig. She was old and ripe, but was very loving and caring. She shielded her from the cold, by finding her a place where the refrigerator blasted the least. She told her stories about her family. She had a daughter just the age of Leek, but sadly she was sold in a different house. Lady Leek reminded the old Fig about her daughter. She showered her with motherly love daily and bit-by-bit, an intimate bond forged amidst them. Leek never had a real mother and was touched by Fig's love. Once again, she rediscovered love. Until one day, the ripe fig was cut open by the beautician to add her juice to a face mask. After that, the ripe fig was left to die; her juices pitifully tripping all over the refrigerator shelf. Once again her faith in humanity was shattered. The days following that particular incident, the beautician decided to re-sell the Leek to a higher bidder. After changing hands many times, Leek finally made it to this house.

Presently, Looking at the smitten couple of Cauliflower and Lady Finger looking into each other's eyes, brimming with love, her heart felt overjoyed once again.

"I am going to make pea soup today from the garden! I hope you eat it! I want no excuses today!" Mum shouted looking over the staircase. The face of all three garden peas in their pod turned pale. Today was their turn to jump in the gunny bag. Others, though felt sorry for garden peas, heaved a sigh of relief for it wasn't their turn to die today.

"No! I hate peas!" Pat came with a grunt from the room upstairs.

"Well, I am making it ditto according to your favourite cookery show." Mum tried to reason.

"I am not going to eat it!" Tee replied poker faced as she bolted down the stairs and headed towards the main door.

"Well, if you eat it! I might allow you to indulge in an ice cream for dessert."

"It's too cold for ice-cream, woman!" Peas screamed silently from the basket, their face contorted in pain. They were going to cry.

The hard expression on the Tee's face softened as she held the main door in her hand .She contemplated the offer once again, "Okay, I guess! Make it delicious!" She shrugged and spoke the last thing before slamming the door shut behind her.

Mum wore the apron again, by tying the flaps on her neck, and switched on the TV. A cookery show was playing on. She removed a notepad and held a pencil in her other hand, to jot down all the ingredients.

"Ladies and gentleman, making pea soup is extremely simple and delicious." The host of the show began talking robotically. "Take a huge bowl; assemble the following ingredients."

Everybody's ears were now pressed to TV; they possibly still might be in danger along with Garden peas.

"You will need Garden Peas, Bitter-Gourd, Cauliflower, Spinach, Leek, skin of lemon for taste and a Lady finger for garnishing.

They all gaped at each other with panic stricken face. Today they were all in a soup, literally. They will be cooked together. It was time, for all of them to jump in the gunny sack to escape their graves.

But Chubby Cauliflower felt more guarded in his hole, after all old habits die hard. He had been hiding in holes since he was a kid.

He looked at Mrs Lady Finger. She too nodded and agreed to hide with him in the small hole at the corner of the top shelve. Even Miss Lady Leek preferred accompanying her friends. Chubby Cauliflower insisted on carrying the baby 'okra'. Mrs Lady Finger couldn't refuse.

They were merely holding their breath for the sheer moment when mommy would be so engrossed in watching the TV that she wouldn't notice them jumping out of vegetable basket and rushing towards their fancied spot.

Currently, she looked at every ingredient on the TV screen and then gazing at them, nodding her head continuously to every word being spoken on TV.

"Mash all the ingredients together in the pan and sauté them in the boiling Water. Add a pinch of turmeric, a bit of pepper and salt to taste. Now put a lid so that………" The host went on. All vegetables glanced at each other. If they don't jump from the basket and run they would all be burning in boiling water.

They impatiently waited for that perfect moment when they could take the plunge. That moment seemed nowhere. Finally lemon tiredly heaved a sigh, and jumped out of the basket. He took the remote lying at a distance on the kitchen counter and pressed few buttons he saw mommy pressing every day.

Mommy rubbed her eyes and wiped her specs. She wondered how the channel got changed automatically. She took the remote and was about to press the back key when she saw the latter channel was playing her favourite series. She forgot to press the previous button and dropped the remote back on the table. The thriller and suspense filled sitcom which also had love, drama and hate immediately engrossed her. It had the perfect ingredients to put her on the edge. She reminded herself to go back to the previous channel and collect the recipe so that her soup would be as perfect as in the cooking show. But after a few moments, she settled down with the idea of downloading the recipe later from the internet. For now she was getting too drawn in her favourite sitcom playing on TV, but not before she noticed a lemon, which had rolled out of the vegetable basket. She picked it up and threw it back in the vegetable basket. She also noticed that all the vegetables were too close to each other and in a perfect proper circle. She broke the circle and placed them at a distance once again. After that her attention was strictly limited to T.V. currently, the hero was going suicidal over his bankruptcy and breakup from his gold-digger girlfriend.

All the vegetables sensed the tension erupting from the small screen and found that to be a perfect opportunity for them to jump from the basket and hide in their hand-picked places. They all hopped and sprinted in their respective direction except Bitter-Gourd. "It's my duty to serve the body, hence I will stay put in the basket only," he quoted like a saint. He grew up in a spiritual environment on the hills of Himalayas besides a temple. He was called the wisest amongst the pack by others, chiefly by the virtue of being the eldest. Spinach and

Lemon ran south towards the gunny bag. The gunny bag was wide open at the foot of kitchen leg. They dived right into few grain particles, which were sitting randomly in it. They preferred gunny bag because it was the most overlooked item in that kitchen. It was merely used to bring grains annually and then went unnoticed throughout the year. All the peas in the pod decided to hop right behind the duo.

Chubby Cauliflower with infant 'okra' cradled in his arms, Mrs Lady Finger and Miss Lady Leek hopped on to climb the wooden cabinets to eventually reach the top shelve. Despite all his chubbiness, Cauliflower showed loads of flexibility while jumping, climbing and most importantly hanging. Hanging where? If one must ask, and then hanging on doorknobs would it be! And can an infant in his arm negate his smooth moves? No, not really. He could do it all with just one hand.

Miss Lady Leek though, was quite lady enough to climb; decided she should blow her etiquettes for a few minutes, given the circumstances. She has been pro at it since at the laboratory where she was born, had many cabinets. She would swing up and down on it all the time until puberty kicked in and her seeds sprouted. Currently, she effortlessly climbed it first to the top shelve, hopping on knob to knob like an athlete. Chubby Cauliflower though swift, was slowed down by inexperienced and amateur Miss Lady Finger. "Sorry", she apologized every time she tripped or stomped her foot on his unintentionally.

And he, like a classic gentleman, gave her his hand at every difficulty and stop, which happened to be a doorknob over here. He too stopped climbing when she was too burnt out to move upwards and couldn't stop panting. He rubbed her back when her breath became heavy and full. He waited for her to recapture it back with lots of compassion in his eyes. He lifted her in his other arm, when it became extremely tricky for her to climb. "Thanks." She whispered in his ears, which sent delightful tingles in his body. He swiftly carried both mother and son to the top shelve. Miss Lady Leek gazed all this from atop. Her heart overwhelmed with emotions. She felt the delicate threads of faith and love sewing themselves back in to her heart. She wished them all the sparks, butterflies and happiness. Eventually, after a heavy climb the two budding love birds and a child joined her at the top. They quickly ran towards the small hole in a corner, which would go unnoticed by mommy, if not gifted with an alert set of eyes.

Commercial time set in and a baby diaper ad broke out. Mommy yawned loudly. She was never this impressed by a mystery in her life.

First, everybody came forward, claiming they had killed the heroine. Be it her gardener, lover, brother, mother, father, and her 7-step sisters. Then, within 24 hours they all took back their claims, saying they were all lying. If this much doesn't get weird, then they had further stumbled upon her 8-step sister. Mommy couldn't wait for the commercial break to get over, so she could further investigate about this new-found 8th step sister. She glanced around the kitchen and found all normal. It was still time before she would start prepping up for her soup. She yawned and stretched a little bit more on the couch.

Another weird claim was being made somewhere up in a hole. "In whichever house I went, I have always found a hole in the wall of the top shelves." Chubby Cauliflower claimed proudly. "In fact, in some houses, I housed in the hole with rodents, bunch of flies, breeds of mosquitoes and strings of spiders." He spoke nostalgic remembering the good times. Though he might be fit now, ironically he was bullied heavily when he was younger for being the clumsiest in the world. "I found my safe heaven in all these holes", He continued, "I escaped into my own world, far away from all the bullies."

While somewhere down south, Spinach, Lemon, Peas and all the grains tried shifting the gunny bag by gunny hoping to a more secluded and isolated place. It was a tiring task since the gunny was obviously too long for their size; and definitely too heavy for their minute hands to hold on to. But spinach was famed for his strength thanks to Popeye and with the help of grains and lemon, they were mightier. They could finally successfully gunny-hop to their new place, while peas cheered for them.

Also the grains, who were all sweet natured and big believers in karma, tried to protect the vegetables by shielding them below. They witnessed the ache on their fellow's grain face, when they were pitifully grinded to powder in the mixer grinder. They were lucky enough to be saved by being overlooked. They were merely retreating the favour now, by giving back to the society, in the form of shielding and protecting the vegetables.

"This is our way of giving back to society. We were extremely lucky!" They said, gratified when vegetables thanked them genuinely.

"It isn't going in the body that is petrifying. I have heard it's a magnificent place! But its burning on flames that scares me to death." Nerdy Spinach Leaf whispered to Lemon, who nodded along in agreement.

"Also, why are humans so ungrateful and waste a good plate of food?" Lemon asked confused.

"They are such idiots." Nerdy Spinach Leaf agreed to Lemon.

"And in carelessness they leave us unattended on high flame and forget everything about us until we are burning black to a crisp." Lemon grunted, "We die an unnatural death."

"My husband died because of heavy burns? Why do they cook us on high flame when we can't handle it?" Mrs Lady Finger cried somewhere up in the north, rocking her son in her arms.

"And we also rapidly lose all our nutrition. The more they burn us in that evil oil and water on high flame, the more we are losing ourselves, our identity and our vitamin." Chubby Cauliflower spoke bitterly while Mrs Lady Finger and Miss Lady Leek nodded their head in agreement.

Chapter 3

Boiling !!!

Swinging over an altitude and watching the antics of vegetables underneath everyday was becoming exhausting and irritating. The bottle of spices, hanging above the kitchen top, rolled their eyes whenever some vegetable or fruit jumped from the basket. No matter how many times and where they hid, they would always be dragged back in the basket and end up in the pot. It was the same old tale! And their conversations were always so boring!

"They have to destroy a nice sunny day by their same old crying. I am so bored." Red-chilli taunted all spiced up.

"They keep bawling that she skinned an Apple. That she is an animal." Pepper cruet rolled her eyes in annoyance. He was just tired of listening to vegetables in the basket for the hundredth time, "Even our people are always treated like that."

"I know right? They keep crying, like we never have to suffer it." Salt bottle huffed back to pepper cruet.

"It's our duty to spice vegetables up. This is what we were born for." Pepper bottle continued.

"Something inside me, tells me that, in some time we all will be brought down." Turmeric bottle spoke psychically.

"Oh your intuitions are always right!" Both Cinnamon and Cardamom bottles turned their attention to turmeric bottle.

"It was nice hanging out with you cardamom." Cinnamon looked in the cardamom's eyes, filled with love.

"Likewise. I love you, Cinnamon."

The show concluded with no fresh twist and turn. Mom stretched her hands and yawned a lot. Who knew watching an intense show could be so tiring. But she had to go back to work before her daughter rang the doorbell. She brought down her bottles of pepper, salt and other spices. She then stood around the vegetable basket and peeked in it. There was nothing in the basket apart from a Bitter-Gourd. She roamed her eye around the kitchen top. Had she even washed and prepared the vegetables for cutting? Or was she merely daydreaming again? She looked around the shelves. Had she or hadn't she? Maybe she needed more coffee.

The cup of coffee lying on the coffee table kept waiting for some more coffee from the jar. Mom poured now cold coffee from the jar into her quarter-filled cup. The cup gulped down the coffee and filled itself to the brim. Jug of water laid by and by besides the cooking stove to add its water when and then called upon by the pan while cooking.

She let off a short sigh of breath and once again cruised back to refrigerator to remove the vegetables. Pitifully, the vegetable compartment in the fridge lay empty. That hinted she had removed the vegetables earlier. Then where were those evil vegetables? This was happening routinely now. Daily some or the other vegetable would disappear and magically appear in some other place. She had to hunt down the whole kitchen to find them. How could she expect today to be any different? Her husband forgot his keys, her daughter refused to eat healthy, the vegetables magically disappeared, and they left the show with suspense again. Routine enough!

"Are there mice in my kitchen?" Mommy panicked at that thought. "Can't be!" she exclaimed. They had just done the costliest pest-control in the home. "What if it flopped?" She worried again. "What if they lay eggs and multiply?" Erg!! Then they would create a storm in the entire kitchen. "What if their kids have already started breeding and multiplying like pigs? Those little rats might be doing all this." This angered her up. She was determined she would search all the drawers and cabinets for mice. She laid down the apron once again on the kitchen top and took a spatula in her hand. "Where are you little runners? You like jogging in my kitchen, don't you? Where are you little rats?" She asked ragingly.

She eye-spied a gunny bag in a dim corner. She did a double take since that was unbelievable. The last time she had checked, the gunny bag was never placed there. She took steps towards the gunny bag. If she had blinked she would have missed the gunny bag moving backwards slightly. But today her eyes were on point and she had not missed the moves made by the gunny bag. That was paranormal! Too bad she was not afraid of ghost!

She opened the gunny bag and found nothing unusual; Apart from few grains tightly sticking to each other over a lemon. She closed the bag. "Wait, what? Over a lemon!" She opened the bag once again and spotted not just a lemon, but surprise-surprise also Spinach and her garden peas underneath the grains. That was funny. She would never place those three in that particular gunny bag. She tried to pull them out. The grains were stuck to each other with an utter terror on their face. They were bonded to each other like glue. They refused to part with each other and definitely refused to let go of the Lemon, Spinach and Peas. They circled them possessively and cemented themselves like a magnet on them. But eventually, after a few minutes of struggle, mommy was finally able to pull Peas, Lemon and Spinach from the grains. After all, how much strength can a tiny dot knock out in front of a giant finger?

"Goodbye, my friends!" The grains whispered sadly to them.

Those three were then rinsed and drained under the sink. All the while, shaking and fumbling as if possessed. She had never seen vegetables moving. Was it healthy to eat moving vegetables? She just shook her head casually when she had no answer and placed them back in the vegetable basket.

She then groped her spatula again and banged opened all the cabinets and then slammed them shut again. She started bashing every shelf with her spatula. Chubby Cauliflower, Mrs Lady Finger and Miss Lady Leek were giving her a tough time in getting caught.

Her eyes caught Lemon rolled out of the basket once more and spinach was just about to hop and garden peas had tripped outside the basket. She threw back the spinach and garden peas inside the basket mercilessly. But she struggled putting the lemon back in the basket. It seemed like he was fighting her hold and kept trying to jump from her clutch. He was extremely unstable below her finger. She somehow with a firm grip placed him back in the basket and placed a lid on them, trapping them inside.

She stood on a stool and looked on the top shelf. Last time when she searched the top shelve, she had caught some Carrot and Radish fantastically making out on the top shelf. Chubby Cauliflower, Mrs Lady Finger, Miss Lady Leek cowered a little lower in their bill. Mommy could have almost missed them, but today her eyes were bang on! Today, nothing could pass by her eyes. She saw lots of green hues in a corner of the wall. Suddenly, she clearly remembered the hole in the corner very well. A Family of rats roomed there once. Once they got rid of it, she completely forgot to seal it. She jumped on the vegetable, but before she could catch them, they skipped out of the hole and jumped into an open drawer. She tried to bang the vegetables in the drawer with her spatula, but they escaped that too. While chubby Cauliflower jumped from one drawer to another, ran from one end of the shelve to another, with infant okra held in his one arm; Miss

Lady Leek and Mrs Lady Finger ran together in another direction. They ran amongst the spoons and plates. A fork even tried to prick them. "Hey!" they screamed at that particular fork. Mommy tried to run behind them, from this end of kitchen to other; alas! They were tad bit too fast for a middle-aged woman.

But nevertheless, mommy was given her chance whenever Miss Lady Leek stopped to help Mrs Lady Finger. Many-a-times Mrs Lady Finger's legs slipped on the slippery coating of china plates. That slowed them down both.

But real table turner was when Mrs Lady Finger hurt her feet at the pointy end of tooth pick and fell down. A little bit of her juice leaked, where the toothpick pierced her leg. Miss Lady Leek also paused her running. Mommy caught them and casted them both in the basket too and closed the lid once again.

"Well, seems she arrested you guys too." Miss Lady Finger stated the obvious, crippling in the basket. Chubby Cauliflower, Nerdy Spinach Leaf and Garden Peas nodded their heads, seated defeated in a corner.

Miss Lady Leek assisted Miss Lady Finger to sit down and tried stopping the leaks from her leg by pressing and covering the wound tightly.

Outside the lid, mommy cursed up a storm under her breath. She seemed determined to catch chubby Cauliflower. She saw a glimpse of green behind a cooker. She held a knife and dived it straight towards that green. She managed to trap his leaves under the knife, a small Lady finger tucked in his arm.

Front door clicked open and the daughter saw her mommy banging the kitchen cabinets, shelves and drawers with her spatula.

Mommy faked a sweet smile as she turned her head and saw her daughter at the door.

"Hello honey! Soup will be ready soon dear!"

Chapter 4

Veggie Talk..!!!

"What's going on? Why are you standing on a stool?" Daughter looked strangely at her mommy.

"Just preparing for the soup!" Mommy spoke in the fake sweet voice.

"Well, I rang the bell and not a soul answered. I had to get the emergency key from the neighbours," daughter spoke further.

"Oh, that's a shame!" Mommy shrugged indifferently.

She picked up the lid and lodged the moving vegetables on the chopping board. She took a razor-edged knife and started cutting the leaves of Cauliflower mercilessly. He screamed and started shaking in pain. But she firmly kept him within her hands as he tried to slip. Other vegetables took a step back in horror, witnessing the spine chilling sight in front of them. They were alarmed of what was going to happen to them next. They looked at each other and shivered.

The Bitter-Gourd cried out a yelp, "You animal," as Mommy cruelly started peeling his skin with a peeler.

Next, she grated the skin of Lemon with a grater. It looked like Lemon had just shaved his head and bottom. While the shaved head looked cool on him. Shaved bottom not so much! She threw him right in the boiling water along with cabbage, gourd and his grated skin though she was not supposed to throw him whole.

"Ouch....you woman!" Lemon screamed from the boiling water of the pot "The cooking show said only skin of lemon. Not full lemon. Are you illiterate?" The lemon kept screaming but his voice was getting mumbled by the hot water. Only bubbles were escaping from his mouth now.

She even separated the three peas from their pod and plunged them all into the boiling water.

She then launched Spinach and Leek right into the boiling water.

She left the pan of boiling water on the stove and let all the vegetable mix in it. The hot boiling water burned all of them. The flame took them over and soon all of them went unconscious.

Lady Finger was witnessing this from the side. She had closed her infant son's eye, who was safely tucked in her arm.

Somewhere after that, even she, and her son were casted on top of the prepared food as garnishee.

>>>>>>>>>>>>>>

Though there was no visible sun, sunlight penetrated deep inside the body through the skin layer. Water washed ashore, and then its waves rippled back into the sea. The sand was made up of rice powder. They say seventy percent of the body is filled up with water. Hence there were bound to be few beaches!

There were herb grasses all over the beach. Tall trees of fruits towered over those grasses. 'If you eat a seed, that seed will grow a tree in your stomach.' One wouldn't know if that was quite true, until that one would witness it themselves. There were beautiful troop of pulpy Beetroots swimming in the sea water, while a bunch of bread loafs lazed around on the sand, soaking up the light. Lust was clear in their eyes as they passed lewd comments on beetroots.

"So moist." A loaf said vulgarly as he saw a young beetroot getting wet in water.

"So fresh and full of juice. I would eat her in a second." His fellow loaf joined him in passing vulgar comments.

"Even you are quite toasty." The young Beetroot flirted back. Both the loaf of Breads started laughing.

The vegetables opened their eyes to beautiful marvels in front of their eyes. They were indeed in paradise. They were experiencing a beach locale. Things which only tropical fruits and vegetables would exclusively experience.

Ambience was breezy and fresh because there was plenty of oxygen in air. Their previous pain of burns was also currently numb, though still a few patches of red and black were quite visible on their skin.

Leaves of chubby Cauliflower were lying detached at a distance. The pod of Peas was not visible anywhere. The last thing that the Peas saw before falling unconscious in pan, was their pod being thrown in dustbin by mommy.

Few powdered skin of Lemon lay there too on sand. "There's your shaved skin. You can glue it back but our pod is gone." One Pea from the trio spoke. "Now, all three of us are separated. We miss bouncing on top of each other." Another two peas nodded in acknowledgement. All three of them looked so similar, that it would be difficult to id them different.

Lemon walked up to his powdered skin. Wherever he stepped, he would leave behind a trail of puss from his shaved skin. He collected the powdered skin in his palms. Same went for Nerdy Spinach Leaf, but it was his specs which lay at a distance. He was provided with specs by his professor, who had grown him organically at his home. Spinach is an excellent source of vitamin A for the eyes; but sadly he himself had weak eyesight, from reading all his professor's books. Bitter-Gourd woke up without his skin, like how mommy had peeled him before putting him in the pan. His skin was missing too, like Peas' pod. "Bet she threw your skin in the bin too." The trio peas told him. "I do not know." Wise Bitter-Gourd replied to them still confused. He was yet trying to make sense of things.

Lady Finger woke up too, but her son was missing. She started fumbling and fidgeting everywhere to find him. Alas! She could not find him anywhere.

"Maa!" a young voice screamed from behind the Herb grasses. She saw a long drumstick carrying her child in her arms, walking through the grass in their direction. Besides Drum-stick, was a long-legged orange Carrot wearing a long green coloured cape and walked with support of a long stick. Behind them were other vegetables of the world like Radish, Broccoli, another long-legged green Chilli, Onion and Potato.

"Welcome to the body!" Long-legged Orange Carrot greeted them cheerfully as they arrived close enough for them to be audible, "Drums honey! Please give the lady her son back."

"Here is your son honey. I found him crying in the shrubs." Drumstick told Mrs Lady Finger kindly.

"And this must be the wonder of the world! So gracious! So beautiful! What a miracle." Carrot praised as he walked up to Miss Lady Leek and kissed her hand; while appraising her from top to bottom.

Miss Lady Leek blushed.

"What a miracle!" He repeated charmingly. "A boon for the world" He added, making Miss Lady Leek blush some more.

"Yes indeed unreal and out of the world!" Lemon sniggered. "She was born in laboratory."

"Don't use that on me." Miss Lady Leek scolded Lemon, "That's racist."

Long-legged Orange Carrot turned around to face every other vegetable which was freshly dropped inside the body.

"I hope you had a pleasant ride, Body can be tricky place." Long-legged Orange spoke coolly.

"We are in the body? I thought we are in Goa or Hawaii." Miss Lady Leek cried disappointed. "People in Britain always ache to go to these places."

"Then where are the humans?" Lemon asked dumbly.

"There are no humans because we are in a human." Mrs Lady Finger said shocked, shocked at his dumbness, ""You are not that bright, aye."

"Lemons are not known to be that bright, because they are sour." Lemon shrugged

"That fails to make sense." Mrs Lady Finger told him off with a straight face.

"And we are in the stomach region to be precise." The Long-legged Orange Carrot continued ignoring their arguments. "We have developed this area to our suitable tastes. We have natural sea and natural waterfalls from the pure mineral water that the girl drinks. We have used rice to make this sand. Behind we have lots of herb grasses. Also there are seeds of fruits scattered all over the stomach. Whenever the girl eats a fruit seed; a plant grows in the stomach." He concluded his long introduction of the place.

"So that fable of "eating a seed will grow a tree" is true?"

"Indeed, it's true! But sadly only for fruits though! Vegetables can be cultivated only by humans and the only way they can enter the body is by being eaten by human!"

"That's very limiting for vegetables!" The fresh stock of vegetables brooded.

"Indeed!" Carrot nodded in agreement, "You had no idea how badly we were waiting for you. Now that you are here, we can gladly transfer the protection of small-intestine to you," he continued.

"The what?" The vegetables asked chorused, their eyes jumped out of their sockets.

"We have been ruling the small intestine from the past two months." The Long-legged Carrot said, indicating towards his team, "but since you all have arrived, it's time for us to sacrifice ourselves in digestion tomorrow and become a nutrient."

"Okay, and?" They all asked, confused.

"And?" He repeated, puzzled, "Oh yes and till the time another capable batch of vegetables are not dropped in the body, you will have to take oath to protect the intestine with all the honesty." He said casually. "Pitifully the northern part of the body like brain is out of our control. So you will have to be extra responsible in protecting the small intestine," he added.

All vegetable looked at each other quizzically. "Why can't fruits do that?"

"Why can't fruits be the protectors?" He repeated absurdly, being thrown off-track with the idea "They are nothing but careless." He laughed off the idea. "They don't do their job well. They are not concerned about the body. They are thieves. They steal nutrients. They are lazy and they refuse to sacrifice themselves for the body. They just want to enjoy till they perish." He ranted suddenly all angry.

Suddenly there was cutting tension in the ambience.

"Where did you get these herb grasses?" Mrs Lady Finger asked trying to flip the cutting tension.

"Oh, we planted them when they came in with the desserts." Long-Legged Orange Carrot said jovially, pleased with the change of subject.

"Tomorrow evening, be your coronation and oath ceremony, immediately preceding which we will sacrifice ourselves." Carrot concluded; but as soon as he saw new vegetables entrant watching the bread loafs lazing around the beach, he immediately added, "You might want to keep an eye for all these bread loafs on the beach. Their king always had flirty eyes for our Beetroots. They might kidnap our red Beetroots again."

He signalled onion and potato poised behind him with his index finger to carry the leaves of chubby Cauliflower.

"We will fix and heal you." He alleged, putting a hand on cauliflower's shoulder. "We have a nursery for healing. There we will glue back your leaves."

"Also, my powdered skin." Lemon added in.

"It would be difficult to glue your powder back, but we will see what we can do." Carrot said thoughtfully, stroking his chin.

"And we have a new range of pods designed exclusively for peas. Also, I am clear, confident about finding a great new skin for Bitter-Gourd from our new market varieties." Long-legged Orange Carrot spoke to peas and Bitter-Gourd. While the Peas were excited, and couldn't wait to bounce on the top of each other; Bitter Gourd didn't seem too excited about the new development.

"That wouldn't be needed. I accept the incident and its scars. I accept my new self the way I am." Bitter-Gourd spoke like a true enlightened saint.

"Impressive!" Long-legged Orange Carrot said charmingly. "Now we should return back to our beautiful homes," he addressed and turned to leave. His team of protectors were following right behind him.

They paced back through the thick grasses. As they journeyed towards the small intestine, they passed by some beautiful garden. A gorgeous, vibrant and brimming with water, waterfall was surrounded with tall and full trees. But what took them aback with their beauty was the blood falls. Red Liquid drops of fall dropped ferociously on the rocks at its bottom. They also crossed the various sizes of tubes and pipes connected to falls.

"You have a lovely home," Miss Lady Leek uttered in wonder, as she took the surrounding in.

"Yes, but now it's yours. We are only guests for a few days. So enjoy while you last!" Long-legged Orange Carrot quoted.

"Our kingdom of small intestine is surrounded by the tubes of large intestine. The Gods have designed it that way and it's very important for our protection. We will take this tube to our home," he said, as they came in contact with a side of a huge rectangular tube. A huge board hung over it which had a large intestine written on it. "This is the large intestine tube." Carrot informed all the fresh vegetables as he turned open a door on the tube. He then asked the new vegetables to step inside it to slide down the tube.

One by one with a slight to-ing and fro-ing the vegetables entered the tube and started sliding down along with Carrot and his team behind. Soon they saw an open door at the other end of the tube. One by one the vegetables started exiting out of that opening. After making sure every vegetable has exited the tube, the Carrot closed that particular door. All the new vegetables stretched their legs from their seventy mini-second ride.

"Welcome to the small intestine." Carrot greeted them as he led them amidst the many small huts lined besides each other. These huts were built from clove sticks and had various doors and windows outlined with leaves. An enormous 3-storey nursery hut stood proudly in the heart of the small intestine.

Whole armies of vegetables and fruits were waiting for them in front of their huts.

Few of the vegetable soldiers had garlands in their hands. As soon as they saw the new troop of vegetables approaching them, they threw the garlands at their neck.

Carrot walked up in the centre, where his throne was placed and clapped for everybody's attention. Even the other protectors, took their thrones besides the carrot.

"Meet your new protectors." Carrot declared. Everybody cheered apart from fruits. They were least interested.

"They will be your new Kings and Queens." There was a shout of hurrah in the small intestine.

"They will be coronated tomorrow," he continued and everybody, apart from fruits and their armies'- clapped .Fruits kept rolling their eyes at every word of Carrot.

"And at first sight of light all the current protectors will sacrifice themselves in digestion to become a nutrient." After the last bit, there was a pin drop silence in the small intestine which was broken by apple.

"Thank god. Finally, the stinking in the stomach will stop." Apple taunted, looking maliciously at Potatoes and Onions. All his fruit girl-friends standing behind started giggling.

Potato and Onion looked down at the bottom of their throne in embarrassment.

"This human will finally stop scaring other humans with her gas leaks," Orange, one of the girlfriend of Apple mocked. At this, the entire fruit army were laughing now.

Potato went red in his face. They were known to create stinky gas in tummy, which sometimes got leaked from the body.

"What a bunch of cruel people!" Mrs Lady Finger whispered to chubby Cauliflower, who was busy ogling at a bunch of beautiful, young red Beetroots.

Mrs Lady Finger ignored and looked away, a tinge of jealously spreading in her heart.

"And the onion will stop leaving that odour in her mouth, which gets on other's nerves." Apple hi -fived his girl-friends now. The whole fruit army were laughing whole-heartedly too. Their laughter echoed through the entire small intestine.

"Well, that's true." Carrot Looked at Onion and Potato disappointedly. "Embarrassing, but true nevertheless; But at least they are ready to sacrifice themselves tomorrow. When will you fruits grow out of being so mean?"

"We might be mean. But you are nothing, but a tall, Long-legged Orange Cartoon." The whole group of fruits was rolling over now from all the amusement.

"That's enough! I exile all of you fruits!" Carrot ordered angrily as he stood up from his throne.

The entire glint from the eyes of fruits disappeared. The fruits and their entire armies looked offended. A frown etched on their faces.

"Fine, we will pack our bags and leave immediately," Apple said scornfully, "But this intestine belongs to us equally."

"I am the king over here. I make the decisions of who belongs here and who doesn't." Long-legged Orange Carrot spoke authoritatively.

"Cool. We will form our own kingdom then in some other organ. We will make it grand and more extravagant than yours." Apple spoke up with all the pride she could muster.

"For that you will have to work hard, which I doubt you will." Carrot shot back at him, "So please excuse me, I have to preside over other important matters."

Apple huffed and turned back to his hut with his girl-friends following him behind. Even the whole fruit army stepped back and decided to decline to their huts, probably to pack their bags.

All the tomatoes looked at each other puzzled. They had a huge identity crisis. The whole world told them they were vegetables. But they always felt like they were fruits. They even had seeds like fruits. Should they stay or should they leave?

One of the Tomato soldiers came forward and declared that all Tomatoes would leave the intestine too, because they were fruits and not vegetable. All the Tomatoes from back nodded and cheered affirmatively, patting the soldier's shoulders. They supported his decision. That made him smile.

Carrot and other vegetables were taken aback by their decision," Are you sure?" He asked them doubtfully.

"Sure as the sun," he told Carrot positively.

"Well! That's a shame! You guys are a bunch of good guys, not careless like fruits; are you still sure?"

The entire fruit army booed carrot for his words, from their hut.

"Positive," tomato soldier spoke with an absolute tone.

The Tomatoes and other fruits hurrahed merrily.

"Suit yourself", the Carrot declared disappointedly.

Long-legged Orange Carrot then turned his attention towards the new stock of vegetables, "So pick up the huts you like. Your respective vegetable army will stay with you," he enlightened them. The new stock of vegetables nodded in understanding.

"So let the preparations for the coronation ceremony begin."

All the seven vegetables entered the 3-storey nursery hut in the heart of the small intestine. Long-legged Orange Carrot led the way inward. Plenty of beds lay there. Many soldiers of vegetable armies were healing the injured soldiers lying on those beds.

His fellow team kings, Potato and Onion, carried the leaves of chubby Cauliflower. They also piled up the powdered skin of lemon that they could accumulate in their fist. "Also, we keep a stock of spare vitamins and minerals. As soon as the body requires it, my trusted army members, send it to that organ via oxygen and the carbon-dioxide trains," Carrot said smiling towards the new stock of vegetables.

"What is oxygen and carbon-dioxide trains?" Lemon whispered to Nerdy spinach leaf.

The leaf of spinach looked back at him in shock. He couldn't believe his ears.

"They are trains." He stated back shocked.

He led them towards a Spinach soldier working in the corner. The soldier looked at the leaves in the hands of Onions and Potatoes and then at the chubby Cauliflower. He quickly nodded as soon as he understood the situation.

"Those leaves are beyond repairs," The Spinach soldier said doubtfully in his rough voice. "I will bring you some lettuce leaves from the store room. They might fit you." He concluded in his rough voice. "Or they might not."

"Lettuce leaves! But I am a Cauliflower," Chubby Cauliflower spoke unbelievably.

"Pardon me. But that's all we have in store room right now." The soldier shrugged as he stood up and went inside the store room at the back. He shuffled around and soon he saw a big pair of Lettuce leaves. He quickly took them in his hands. Also, when he saw the glue lying on the grounds, he grasped that quickly too. While he held glue in one hand, he came out of the store room along with a big pair of Lettuce leaves fastened in his other hand.

When chubby Cauliflower saw the leaves he gulped, "This leaves are too big. They would get stuck everywhere," he whined. Spinach soldier just shrugged at that. Chubby Cauliflower looked at his fellow vegetables. Even they just shrugged. Nobody cared.

Eventually the Lettuce leaves were stuck to the chubby Cauliflower's body. He looked funny because the leaves were bigger than his body.

Something in the other corner caught the trio Peas' attention. They hopped towards it.

Potato then transferred the skin powder of Lemon to the Spinach soldier. The soldier then pasted some sticky glue on the round bottom of Lemon, from where some of his skin was shaved. He stuck all the powder to his round bottom, leaving none for his head. Also, the powder was stuck unevenly, leaving few spots thinly covered with powder. The puss would still leak from there.

"Hey!" he busted outrageously, "That's a dirty work you did there!"

Spinach soldier just shrugged.

"And you left none for my head."

"Well that's good because your shaved head looks trendy," Miss Lady Leek appraised him.

Those words of Lady Leek boosted the confidence of Lemon and he felt much better.

"If you want, I have some hand-made leave hats in the store room, which you can wear." Before Lemon could answer, the soldier went back to the store room and arrived with few leave hats. "Try them in your hut," he instructed Lemon.

Later he asked Bitter-Gourd, if he would like to try their "new in the market" skins, which Bitter-Gourd politely declined.

In the other corner of the hut the Peas were having the time of their life. They had never seen so many bright pods in their life. They thought pods came only in one colour, "green". But here there were pink, orange, white, black and all the rainbow colours.

"You have a beautiful collection!" They asserted in awe.

"We dye normal pods with food colours which of course comes with food," the Carrot soldier who was entertaining them spoke.

"Yes, we have heard about it! They add it in food in restaurants." They acknowledged the fact and the soldier nodded along.

All Peas climbed on each other to try the pods.

"We will start with the yellow. It's vibrant," the bottom Pea suggested.

"But I want glamorous. Black is glamorous." The middle one disagreed with bottom one.

"I want chic. Let's go with blue." The top one belted out its two cents.

****

A young and fresh Beetroot knocked twice on the semi-open door of a hut. An army of Cauliflowers lived in that hut. Some came with pizza while other came with the burger. Hence the majority of them were solidly soaked in oil. The oil made them slow in movement; hence she bumped into several of them while finding her favourite Cauliflower. Though chubby, he was hands down the fittest vegetable in the whole intestine. Her ex-banana was all body and no brain. He was also a double-dater. Chubby Cauliflower was Cherry on top; intelligent too, after all he was going to be their new king. Of course, she meant the cherry of the idiom; Not her friend Cherry. She would never let her friend Cherry talk to him.

She had to break up with Banana because their paths were getting separate. He along with other fruits was leaving the intestine to live in some other organ. It was a sad farewell because good-byes were always sad. But it wasn't that sad since he was two-timing her with Strawberry.

He always claimed their red colour confused him. How would that be possible? Because while she was maroon red, Strawberry was passion red; He was lying. Then chubby Cauliflower caught her eyes. The old spinach soldier was gluing him lettuce leaves in the nursery, though they looked a tad bit odd on him, he looked handsome never-the-less. And course he was smart, since he was going to be their new crowned king.

"Your hair looks amazingly parted," She cooed when she saw him combing his hair with his hand.

She caught him off-guard. Her beauty stunned him like a deer caught in headlights. He froze, inept to speak for a few minutes. "Than..nkks," he stumbled. "You look umm, am-amazing too."

"Lemme be your date to the coronation," she lipped.

"Okay," he replied, stunned.

In the adjacent hut, Mrs Lady Finger was busy tucking her crying infant in bed. All the new places made him cry. Whilst he was getting accustomed to the kitchen, they were eaten inside the body. Though she was stressed over her crying baby, she couldn't wait to see chubby Cauliflower tonight and have some private intimate time with him. In some other hut, Lemon was trying different leaves to cover his thin skin patches. His puss was trailing from thin patch everywhere he walked. While Bitter-Gourd was resting and recouping himself for the big coronation event in his hut, Miss Lady Leek in opposite hut was peeping outside her window at the decorations. There were seven new thrones being decorated with leaves and flowers. Inside the hut, her army, who insisted Lady Leek to call them her 'fans', apparently they had spent too much time with fruits, finished getting her a floral and leaf dress. She saw them with a tinge of dreamy eyes. They were so real. Real body! Real soul. While she was 'soo…' artificial! And they called her a miracle. Her! That was pathetic! They all were the real and natural miracle.

Meanwhile, garden Peas were still trying on various new and glamorous pods from the nursery. They still couldn't decide which was the most vibrant, glamorous and chic pod. They finally settled on an orange pod with a yellow lily drawn on the back of the pod. The Carrot soldier, who doubled up as personal shopper for them, was only happy to help them to put it on.

King Carrot looked at the decorated thrones and seemed impressed. Behind him were his team of fellow protectors and his entire vegetable army. Also standing at backdrop were now few abandoned huts after the fruits and their armies left them.

As soon as vegetables made their entry they all clapped. First entered the chubby Cauliflower, with his plus one, the pulpy, fresh and juicy Beetroot. At that time, he had completely forgotten about Mrs Lady Finger; He was then followed by lemon and garden peas rolling and hopping behind him. Mrs Lady Finger and Miss Lady Leek came in together next, hand-in-hand. Mrs Lady Finger's heart froze when she saw Beetroot and chubby Cauliflower flirting. She decided to spend the entire evening with Miss Lady Leek and try to keep a safe distance between them. Bitter-Gourd entered last.

The coronation ceremony commenced as Carrot asked them to take the oath. "We will protect the intestine from King Bread, infections and injuries. We will heal the body. We will strengthen the bones and when the right time comes we will sacrifice our-self to become nutrients."

After Long-legged Orange Carrot being satisfied with the oath, they took the throne and sat on it proudly. Armies marched forward and saluted them. But after some to-ing and fro-ing and few hush-hush internal discussions, the new king and queen decided to get up from the throne and decline it. They addressed everyone that they would protect the small intestine without a throne.

Everybody cheered and clapped. Delightful whistle boomed throughout the intestine, after all their new king and queen had not only been coronated; but they were as humble as soil.

Feasting of organic soil and fertilizers soon followed the coronation. Beetroots and chubby Cauliflower danced salsa together, while Mrs Lady Finger and Miss Lady Leek did their chic dance. Lemon and garden Peas just hopped and rolled around and wise, Bitter-Gourd clapped from the side.

The coronation ceremony went on throughout the night, but as soon as the light's first ray broke through the skin, Carrot and the other older king and queen knew it was time for them to walk down the digestive track.

With sad, gloomy and down casted eyes, they all walked towards the digestion. Everybody followed them sadly. Before entering it, they bid goodbye and wished the new protectors all the luck.

Chapter 5

We are the healers

A black, yucky smelling and disgusting looking egg tumbled through the tubes of large intestine like a ping pong ball in a computer game. A zoo of micro-organisms was buzzing on its head.

Eventually, it landed with a "thud" on the grounds at the entrance of the small intestine.

Every vegetable left their huts in curiosity. They pondered over the egg in a fashionable excitement. This kind of egg had never been sighted before in the entire body.

'Oh praise the lord! Finally, something besides bread.' garden peas exclaimed thrilled.

"And big and round," Miss Lady Leek clapped her hands, echoing a delight similar to that of garden peas.

"And stinky and disgusting", Apple taunted from the corner, standing with his girlfriends.

"O hush-hush! Don't be such a mood buster now!" Mrs Lady Finger scolded.

"I bet from the stinky smell, that it's a potato", Apple snapped back.

"Well, that would be nutritive for the body. Rich in vitamin c, b, ir....." The Nerdy Spinach Leaf started ranting from the side.

"Yeah...stop!" All the fruits stopped spinach right in middle of his rant.

"Hurray! Good news!" all the vegetables jumped with happiness.

"O hell! Whole stomach and intestine is going to stink now. I can already smell all the gases," Strawberry flipped with disgust. "And it doesn't even look like a potato," she rolled her eyes.

"I hope it gets digested quickly." Cranberry as she covered her nose with her hands.

"Mommy, what is digestion?" Baby Lady Finger named 'okra' by his late dad, Mr Lady Finger asked, tucking at his mommy's skirt.

"You die!" Apple laughed evilly.

"No!" Mommy Lady Finger busted, disturbed at what her little boy just heard. "We just get transformed into nutrient," she spoke hastily trying to redeem the situation. Chubby Cauliflower placed his hands on twice his length, Mrs Lady Finger's shoulder.

"Why are you even here? Aren't all fruits exiled form small intestine?" Miss Lady Leek asked apple distastefully.

"True, we are! But I am here to see and collect if any fruit drops in the small intestine," Apple spoke casually.

"But, when did Potatoes skin start coming in black?" Lemon wondered in amazement standing beside the Nerdy Spinach Leaf. "It looks glamorous though. I like this new Potato."

Disappointment swept through the entire small intestine when they realised Potatoes are yellow not black. All cheering and clapping stopped.

"O hush! Hush, it's a new technology," Cubby Cauliflower said coolly.

"Tanning Booth", Strawberry opined. Apple looked at her sternly.

"Or perhaps it's that new science breakthrough invention they were talking about, the one that is hybrid of potato and grape," Nerdy Spinach Leaf suggested.

"Wow! That makes sense!" Lady Leek said in a delightful relief.

"I like the new hybrid Potato," Lemon said flirtingly.

"Oh really? So you are confident that humans who never eat real fruits and vegetables are now eating the hybrid ones," Apple taunted back "You people are so dumb. You will never learn now, will you?"

"Why do you always have to speak so nasty? Maybe they finally started appreciating us." Mrs. Lady Finger said hopefully.

"O fool! Go ahead and be innocent! But this will never be true.

Who really saves them?

Batman.

That spider bitten Spiderman,

Or that stud harry potter.

It's us and it has always been us

The Healers

But they will never worship us. They will never make a movie on us or run behind us screaming our name."

Apple Swore loudly.

"That's might be true. But let's not forget we were born to protect them and we will die only protecting them. It's our duty," the wise, Bitter-Gourd spoke calmly.

"You vegetables can do whatever you want. But we fruits will never follow this madness." Apple spoke acidly.

"But you cannot let one incident scare you from doing your duty." The wise Bitter-Gourd declared.

"One incident?" Apple spoke unbelievably, pushing away all the memories of that day "We heal them all the time and that nasty laboratory medicines sweeps away all our credit," Apple blinked back the tears threatening to break loose.

That day still gave him goose-bumps. The girl had developed acidity in stomach. And the hot acid lava from the volcano had almost burned his skin. He had fainted after exerting all his juices trying to calm down the volcano.

He was chilling in the tall herb grasses near the waterfall in the stomach when the smoke started to rise in the entire region. The air had become hot and dense. A burning sensation passed through the air and started moving towards the chest. "It's Acid" Apple warned everybody nearby.

Immediately Apple gathered his army of Apples and started a journey towards the volcano to calm it down.

He jumped right into it. His entire skin started turning black. He collapsed. Even most of his soldiers had jumped into the acid volcano. He lost most of them right in front of his eyes. Medicines arrived much later; after the show ended, to be precise.

But for months after that, medicines were dropped periodically in the intestine. But alas! There was no new sign of any Apples in the intestine. "Once again medicines were preferred," Apple continued in an angry tone. He still had black scars from that day.

Everybody had a pity look on their face.

"Happens what may, we must still do our duty," wise Bitter-Gourd once again came forward to speak. "We will be appreciated one day. Our fruits of labour will be rewa……"

"Everybody might want to step back," Nerdy Spinach Leaf said gazing the egg analytically, "I am afraid this is no potato."

And true to his words the black egg started Jiggling and shaking. Everybody stepped back in fright. The egg hatched and a black worm popped out of it.

Strawberry was the first one to scream, Banana, who was busy flexing his muscles, screamed second. Apple's eyes widened and the Peas shoved themselves back in their pods.

Panic arose and stampede broke as everybody started running to and fro.

The Worm climbed down the egg and started wiggling in random directions.

"Incoming," chubby Cauliflower shouted like a true hero on a bike. He zoomed his bike in the air over the black Worm, which was now moving towards their huts.

Both the pulpy Beetroot and Mrs Lady Finger looked at him in awe. He looked like a real warrior when he took out a knife and threw it at the Worm.

****

"I think so, I am not that sure," Tee told the doctor again and again. "My friend started freaking out when she saw a black egg in her water. And I fear I drank it too, since we both filled our bottles from the same water tap."

"Oh! Do not worry darling, Just take these medicines and all worms in your stomach will die," Doctor said smoothly.

"Are you sure I will have to take these?" Tee asked cautiously. Her cabinet was overflowing with medicines. She was already taking medicines for digestion, acidity, leg pain, head and stomach aches and, now, worms! Her friends already teased her, patient and ambulance, and how she always made them feel right at hospital.

"Do not worry, Sweetheart! Medicines and tablets are our best friends," Doctor smiled brightly.

Chapter 6

The fable.

An old folk's fable:

Bread will rise up one day;

in not too distant future,

and slaughter all the descendants of vegetables and fruits.

Nerdy Spinach Leaf made his way through the herb grasses. The beach was filled with crumbs of bread crashed on the rice sand. He huffed in disgust seeing their fatty acids spilling out of their bodies.

"Gross! Littering the beach! Lowlife hooligans!"

He walked through the herb grasses towards the waterfall and stood on a water pipe.

"Census time." he shouted. "All the protectors bring your freshly arrived armies. It's census time." His voice boomed throughout the small intestine.

All pack of army leaders left their huts, each with their entire newly-arrived pack of soldiers. They marched in troops one behind the other and aligned themselves near the waterfall.

"Very Well then," Nerdy Spinach Leaf appraised, opening his register memo. "Let's begin the census."

He jumped from the pipe and walked up to the first troop of vegetable. The troop of Tomatoes!

The army leader stepped aside and a bunch of new soldiers stepped ahead.

Nerdy Spinach Leaf looked them upside-down and frowned, "too old and rotting. What brought you all?"

"A stale pizza." all soldiers answered in weak and feeble voices.

"You have no juice, seems like you were crushed in heavy oil."

"A low quality, Not fit for Battle."

Tag was placed on their heads.

Nerdy Spinach Leaf wore a tear protection mask before moving to the next troop, a troop of Onions.

Spinach judged them from top to bottom. “Strong, sharp and tough, perfect for cold”, a “Fit for Battle” tag was placed on their head tips.

Next was a troop of Lemons. Nerdy Spinach Leaf almost tripped on their puss. “Acidic, stingy, will do fine….,” an “Acceptable tag” was hanged on their bellies.

Next was a troop of Broccolis “Came with stale pizza again.” Low quality, semi decayed, though not fully rotten yet.” “Acceptable for Battle” tag was placed on their necks.

“AHH, brothers,” Nerdy Spinach Leaf exclaimed when he saw that next was a Troop of Spinaches.’

“Burger brought them here,” the leader Spinach stated, “But they are as fit as horses.”

“Acceptable for Battle” tag hung on them without even checking their conditions.

Next troop was a Bunch of ‘Lettuces’ which had come with salad. Salads were always healthy; hence Spinach placed an “accepted for battle” on their thin leaves even without a thought.

Next troops were of Carrots and Radish. They were old friends of Spinach’s. “An accepted for battle tag,” was thrown in their tiny neck without any further inquiry.

“Next troop is Beetroots,” Nerdy Spinach Leaf muttered under his breath looking at his paper when he moved forward, but frowned when he came face-to-face with a troop of Garlic instead of Beetroots. He pushed back his glasses which had flown down his nose. “Are you the new hybrid Beetroots?” He inquired.

“Huh?!”Garlics raised their eyebrows in confusion.

“The ones who were supposed to have the colour of Radish, but had to be Beetroots,” Nerdy Spinach Leaf mumbled.

“No! We are Garlics,” the Garlic leader voiced.

“Then where are Beetroots?” Nerdy Spinach Leaf asked confused.

“I don’t know,” the Garlic leader mumbled.

“But you live right in the adjacent hut?” Nerdy Spinach Leaf asked again alarmed.

“I don’t know.”

Nerdy Spinach Leaf sighed irritatingly.

"Beetroot army have disappeared in thin air." A baby Garlic came forward and made public his information. "I had last seen them taking a bath in this waterfall at dawn. They never returned back to their huts." baby Garlic spilled, pointing towards the water-fall behind them.

"Aga-a-a-in?" Nerdy Spinach Leaf drawled, trying to process this new piece of information.

Baby Garlic looked confused.

Nerdy Spinach Leaf looked doubtfully towards the bread crumbs lounging on the beach in the distance through herb grasses. Anger rose in him. The crumbs crawled down a little lower, hiding themselves behind the grasses to avoid his murderous gaze.

"It's the king bread again, isn't it?" Nerdy Spinach Leaf asked the Wise Bitter-Gourd, who was standing just behind him. Wise Bitter-Gourd nodded.

"King Bread kidnapped Beetroots right under our nose, again!" Miss Lady Leek exclaimed unbelievably.

"As protectors of small intestine, our power has been tested again." Lemon cried defeated "and once again we fail."

"Pardon me, sir, but what do you mean by again? How many times has it happened before?" Baby Garlic asked confused.

"Once. She was a heavenly attractive woman, brimming with youth!" Chubby Cauliflower said dreamily. "She was graced with every quality a Beetroot should be blessed with."

"What happened then?" Baby Garlic asked with curiosity.

"It was dawn on that gloomy day too, when Beetroot went for a bath in this very same waterfall." Chubby Cauliflower stressed, pointing towards the waterfall behind him. "On that day too she was looking devastatingly beautiful in her red bikini. Like the most beautiful woman on earth that she is! She was humming as usual, in her beautiful sing-a-song voice. She emerged out of falls, water dripping from her hair and body, her cheeks redder than ever, her curves curvier than ever. She was glowing!" Chubby Cauliflower continued, stressing on each word passionately. "Beetroots are known for their reddest skin in the world. But her blush was most luminescent, like never seen before!" Then his face turned thunderous with anger. "She caught the fancy of king bread, who was driving pass the waterfall in his Porsche. In that spit-second, king bread developed a crazy love for her. He asked his guards to kidnap her in a hurry. That was the last time she had been spotted," cubby Cauliflower concluded his sad story with tears in his eyes.

"And this time, he dared to abduct the whole, freshly arrived army." Lemon voiced infuriated.

"Sir, I am afraid, it's the whole army and not just the freshly arrived," baby Garlic uttered the words in terror, "There is nobody in their hut," he continued looking at everybody's thunderous faces.

"Perhaps the legendary fable of bread imprisoning us in the toilet jail and eventually flushing us out of the body is coming true," Nerdy Spinach Leaf stated.

Mrs Lady Finger covered her baby's ears, while chubby Cauliflower pulled her closer towards her and caressed her arms soothingly.

"OMG! We are doomed!" Miss Lady Leek cried.

"Don't be silly. We are the Protectors of the small intestine. Our army will break their spines on our commands. The Fable is a merely a fairy tale," Lemon spoke proudly.

"But King bread has already captured the whole brain. He has even set up his throne at the 'desire point', the point from where he controls the desires of entire body. Perhaps at the moment that's where our Beetroots' are," Nerdy Spinach Leaf stated.

"OMG! We are doomed!" Miss Lady Leek cried again.

"Then we will go to desire point in the brain and bring our Beetroots' back. They are not just soldiers, but also our family," the wise, Bitter-Gourd spoke calmly yet determined.

"Then it's done. Tomorrow at first sight of light, we protectors will leave for desire point in the brain and return only with Beetroots." Lemon declared.

Everybody cheered.

Tee looked down at her weighing scale disappointedly. Her mommy had told her that exercising will reduce her weight. So, the past whole week, every morning, she had dragged herself from the bed. Granted initially she used to switch off the alarm and snoozed back to sleep. But then every night she started placing her favourite model's picture next to her pillow, to give herself much needed will power. She walked a little bit on the first day, a little bit more on the second day and a lot more on the remaining days. Her legs were tired, but she stood excitedly on the weighing scale nevertheless, until she looked down. Two pounds more. Her mouth fell down to the ground in shock.

"Congratulations honey! That's your muscles increasing their weight. You are on the right track," mommy excitedly thumped the girl's back in encouragement and went back to her work.

"But aren't they supposed to lose their weight," the girl muttered under her breath with a straight face to no one in particular.

Chapter 7

Human Atlas.

It was midnight. The room was dark black. Chubby Cauliflower kept flicking the switch of lamp continuously in hopes that electricity will start burning and room will be filled with light again. "Cells don't produce electricity in sleep." Nerdy Spinach Leaf hissed at his lack of ignorance. "We will have to read maps in dark black only," he spoke casually. "Well easy for you to say mate. Spinaches can see in the dark because of vitamin A. What about us?" Lemon huffed as he squinted his eye to try and analyse the map. A human atlas was laid wide open on table. Everybody gathered around it.

"There are two routes that we can use to reach the brain. First is the digestive route passing through stomach- throat – nose and second route is a circulatory system via the lungs and heart," Spinach stated clearly.

"The first route is out of option. If we get stuck in the throat, the girl will vomit us out of the body." Bitter- Gourd brooded.

"Hmmm", chubby Cauliflower agreed, "Then we have no choice but to take route 2."

"Very well, then! But I must warn you beforehand, we will have to take a carbon-dioxide train till lung station, " Nerdy Spinach Leaf spoke swiftly.

Everyone's face lost colour, "are you trying to say we will have to take a carbon-dioxide train till lung station?" Miss Lady Leek asked scared.

"I am afraid so! That is exactly what I am saying," Spinach nodded at everyone "We can take an oxygen train to brain only after changing trains at lung station."

"Monster carbon dioxide and the blue blood!" Miss Lady Leek screeched dramatically, "that's like opening a trouble box. We can never survive that."

"That's nonsense! We will die like rotten Tomato in carbon-dioxide train!" Lemon exclaimed looking horrified.

"Let's go back to discussing route one then," Lemon said nodding his head dismissively.

"That would be worse, if the girl vomits us, how are we supposed to then bring back the Beetroots?" Chubby Cauliflower argued.

The wise, Bitter-Gourd who was listening silently till now spoke up, "It's true, we will have to adjust our journey till lung organ by travelling in carbon-dioxide train only."

"Oh my my! Miss Lady Leek exclaimed, "We are all going to die a brutal death, aren't we?"

"I am more concerned about the well-being of my little boy. Hope he doesn't cry too much in my absence. That would be such a shame on me!" Mrs Lady Finger sobbed and then cleared her throaty throat. She had just joined them after tucking her little boy in bed, who she would be leaving behind in protection of her Lady-Finger armies. "This would be the first time my little boy is being separated from me. First his dad; now me, such a shame on me!" She sniffed loudly.

"Don't be afraid my lady. The boy will be only more cherished and loved in your absence," Chubby Cauliflower whispered soothingly in her ears, tucking a loose strand behind her ear.

"Hope so," Mrs Lady Finger said weakly.

****

Tee's mom scolded her for the hundredth time. "Learn to accept yourself. You should love your body the way it is." But can she? Her friends would laugh at her if she told them she was happy with her body. They would just tease her that she looked like a skirt from her waist. There was no one who resembled her on television. If models were fat then nobody would watch TV, at least that's what her friends told her. "Fine, if you want to improve the way you look then try to be active. Stay fit, don't be on couch whole day." Her mom advised her after she was constantly crying. "But that's not helping me either. Exercise is increasing my weight" Tee whimpered back, "I just want to be like models. My friends say Model's don't eat. Probably I should try that." Hearing that Tee's mom placed her hands on her hips sternly, "You are trying no such nonsense." She said firmly, "Not eating doesn't solve anything. Doesn't make you feel good. Exercise takes time. But it will show results."

Mrs Lady Finger kissed her son "goodbye", Nerdy Spinach Leaf tucked the map under his arms, garden Peas wore their new set of fashionable pod, and Lemon washed his hut from the puss he had leaked the entire night. Bitter-Gourd and Spinach Leaf instructed their armies to protect the small intestine in their absence. Cauliflower couldn't stop brushing his hair. He wanted them to be as neat as possible to dazzle away Mrs Lady Finger off her feet. 'Score', He hi-fived himself in the mirror after he was pleased with the way he looked.

As the first sight of light broke through the skin, all protectors came out of their huts. They marched towards the station, putting one foot ahead of another, singing songs of courage, glory and victory.

We are heroic to erect your spine,

We are cloth to wash your stomach,

We have guts to strengthen your guts,

We are saviours to save your heart,

Victory is our middle name

Nobody heals better than us.

La-la-la-la-la-la-la-la-la

Because we are a something great to hold on to,

To have a long life,

We destroy ourselves to create you,

Eat, drink or churn us in your mixer,

We are all yours.

La-la-la-la-la-la-la

"Okay, troop of singing idols, you all are forbidden to go any further without a ticket," a barrier spoke at the entrance of the station. He was busy smoking from a small pipe.

"Tickets?" chubby Cauliflower asked dumbly.

"Yes, can I please see your tickets?" The barrier squeaked again.

Everyone turned their heads to glare at Spinach Leaf. He was the one, who was the knowledgeable amongst them.

"Digestive route doesn't ask for a ticket," Nerdy Spinach Leaf spoke casually.

"That's because the digestive route has no organised system. Any tom, dick and harry can just hop on it. No wonder half of the human race has the stomach ache and the other half is always puking." barrier laughed, "But circulatory system is a sophisticated system. If you are a nutrient, the ticket counter will issue you a ticket itself."

"Of course, the body requires us. We need to bring back the Beetroots from the brain. We need Beetroots to fulfil the needs of the body." Chubby Cauliflower tried to be reasonable.

"Then you better get going by a car, because to board the train you need to have a ticket. To have a ticket you have to be a nutrient which you all are not," barrier suggested while smoking his pipe.

"A car? A car you say," Miss Lady Leek busted angrily, placing her hands on her hips firmly. "Do you have any idea how much pollution a car causes? If you are ignorant, Nerdy Spinach Leaf can enlighten you," she screamed at the red jelly.

"A lot of amount, a car takes in lots of oxygen and gives out a lot of carbon-dioxide which is harmful for body," Nerdy Spinach Leaf spoke immediately.

"Is that what you desire? To give harmful carbon-dioxide to the body, or to use up all the oxygen in the body," Miss Lady Leek barked at barrier, smoke coming out of her ears.

"No not really. That would be devastating!" barrier bit back its tongue.

"Clearly, now point us to the ticket counter," she demanded.

The barrier pointed them towards a machine standing on a podium and all the vegetables walked towards it to issue themselves a ticket.

****

Bloated, she felt. Guilty, she felt. The remorse was making her heart sad. One more failure in her efforts. An hour back while coming back home, she tried so hard to look away from the billboard covered with the giant pizza. She could smell the delicious melted cheese from it. Now all her head could think was ways of eating that gorgeous pizza sitting in her refrigerator when she reached home. Whole day she had ignored all the painful hunger in her stomach. Her mom was pretty angry when she refused to have her lunch. That thunderous sound of hunger in her stomach was embarrassing to say the least. She had held herself up, pretty well till now. She had even congratulated herself for not letting even a single food particle enter her mouth. But night is when, all her will power crumbled down. Plus, this pretty Instagram worthy picture was doing no justice to her determination. Once home, she couldn't stop her hands from grabbing that particular pizza from the refrigerator, a leftover burger in oven and a coke. After guffawing everything down, she just felt bloated and incredibly guilty. From tomorrow, for sure, she would sincerely not eat anything.

Chapter 8

Monsters!!!!!!!!!!

There is magic in veins they say.

But alas! There is no magic in veins!

There are only monsters in veins. But if one has to turn everything poetic, try artery!

All the vegetables made a line for their turn on the machine. Currently a family of zinc were engrossed in scanning the vitals of their newly-born. A card zoomed out from the machine.

Level:-developing.

Final Destination:-facial skin.

Designation: - fight the bacteria's of acne.

"Weee," The new-born clapped delighted, happy with his position and the family stepped down from the podium.

"Now it's my turn," Lemon declared as he bounced himself on the podium. He pressed the blue button on the machine and a round image of Lemon popped on the screen.

"I look like a tennis ball," Lemon wondered.

"A yellow tennis ball, I presume," a garden Pea said, "Green would look something like our skin." All the other peas in pod bounced up and down in agreement.

Without warning, the machine beeped and a 'No nutrient', sign was displayed in bold letters on the screen of the machine.

"No nutrient, but I am full of vitamin C!" Lemon exclaimed bluntly, "This machine is quite useless."

"Maybe because it's not visible", Miss Lady Leek uttered, "otherwise it would have issued you a ticket."

"Visible?" Lemon asked. Chubby Cauliflower nodded his head. "We can make our nutrient visible."

"Aye" Nerdy Spinach Leaf asserted. "This calcium knife might work." He walked up to a knife placed in its holder and dislodged it from its holder.

"Oh that would probably be an excellent idea," Chubby Cauliflower nodded impressed.

"Make my vitamin C visible with it then. Bring my flesh out," Lemon voiced boldly.

Spinach blew a hit on his head with the knife. Puss oozed out from the fresh crack that had been developed by the blow.

"Is my nutrient visible?" Lemon asked in a pained voice, trying to tolerate the sharp pain that had just tingled his body from the blow.

"Not even close. Your juice is not dripping properly yet," Spinach said confused.

"That's going to be very slippery," Chubby Cauliflower grimed.

"Also messy and dirty". Barrier shouted. His patience was being tested by the idiotic actions of the vegetables. He made an extreme irritated face.

"Try it on me bud," chubby Cauliflower participated.

"Alright" Spinach spoke casually and hit the knife on chubby Cauliflower's belly, breaking one of his lettuce leaves.

"Ouch," chubby Cauliflower yelped as it fell down on floor in pain, "that's painful."

"Okay, you illiterates!" Barrier spoke in an irritated voice, "That's enough stupidity for today."

A family of amino acids was passing by the barrier. He stole their cards from their backpack.

"Hey. But we have to go to work," the acids cried.

"Yeah, you can die some other day," barrier answered back harshly.

"This is so horrible." Tee was suffering from an all-time low self-esteem. Her self-esteem had taken a major hit. Her plan to not eat only made her fight of losing weight more difficult. Every morning she would promise herself not to eat, but at night her urge to eat would become uncontrollable and she would end up eating all the fattening foods she could find at a sensational speed. Nights made her weak. Her hunger intensified at night after not eating the whole day. She kept scolding herself for giving into the pressure of hunger every night. Her guilt was eating her soul. She cried herself to sleep every night. Not eating throughout the day and eating at night was adding more kilos to her existing kilos. With a heavy heart, puffy eyes and a bloated body, she chucked the idea of crash diet out of the window because it just wasn't working.

After profusely thanking the barrier, all the vegetables proceeded towards the carbon-dioxide train, which would arrive at platform number three. They walked their way through all the hustle and bustle of the platform number one. It was bustling with activities. Though it was incredibly crowed, everything was organised. All the nutrients had queued up graciously for their turn to climb up the oxygen train when it would arrive. Soon a train arrived on the platform number one and a fresh batch of oxygen bubbles climbed down from it. Those bubbles were bouncing electrifyingly.

"I wish even we could go in oxygen train instead of carbon-dioxide train," Mrs Lady Finger wished hopefully. "But, my dear lady that train won't take us to our destination. We can't climb that," chubby Cauliflower rubbed his hands on her.

Next a family of vitamin C descended from oxygen train, "look that family is formed from my ancestor's puss," Vitamin C spoke excitedly. Everybody congratulated him on his back.

A bunch of jumpy glucoses jumped off the train. Another barrier was trying to calm down that bunch of jumpy glucoses. It was day time and they had assumed that even today the human won't eat anything throughout the day. Hence the small intestine had ordered extra bunch of glucose just in-case.

After all the nutrients from the train had climbed down, all the nutrients in que then climbed up the train and many of them took the window seat.

The aura was all fresh on platform number one.

But platform number three was a complete contrast to platform number one. The ambience of the platform three was dark and gloomy. It was suffocating from the lack of oxygen. As soon as they reached that platform, random white and yellow stones started attacking them.

"Stones." Lemon shouted excitedly when he saw them.

Mrs. Lady Finger, let out a sharp cry as a tiny yellow stony tried to block her way. The stone grinned evilly at her. Chubby Cauliflower placed his arms around Mrs Lady Finger "Do not be scared. They won't do anything apart from blocking and smiling creepily at you." But he spoke too soon as a yellow stone pounced on him and punched him on his face.

"Go way you creep," Nerdy Spinach Leaf stabbed a huge stone with the knife he had gotten at the ticket machine. He kept with himself because he figured he might need it.

"OO and sometimes they might try and eat you too," Lemon told Mrs Lady Finger casually. Lady finger shivered hearing that, "But not me. My puss is too acidic for them." He smiled at her warmly as he continued scaring her unintentionally. "Even him." Lemon pointed towards the Bitter-Gourd, who was walking ahead of them. "His bitterness is too bitter. Stones don't really like it." Lemon whispered to Mrs Lady Finger.

Garden peas punched a few stones themselves. Two of those stones attacked the Chubby Cauliflower again from behind, but garden peas picked them and smashed them with each other.

A cluster of blue blood bubbles flowing in the corner laughed loudly at their misery.

A carbon-dioxide train soon arrived on the platform number three. "Here quick" Bitter Gourd punched the tickets in the ticket slot and the train compartment door opened up. Everybody ran and rushed inside the train. They all leaned against the train wall for support, tired from their sudden run.

"That was nasty. That thing almost bit me," chubby Cauliflower muttered under his breath.

"And little bit of my pod broke off trying to kick those rocks," Lady Peas complained.

"Thank you for protecting me," Mrs Lady Finger said shyly to chubby Cauliflower.

"It was an honour," Chubby Cauliflower bowed.

There was a faint voice coming from inside the train chamber. The faint voice became louder as they opened the door of the chamber.

The train chamber was filled with blue blood bubbles and large cubes of sugar and salt. They made their way towards the window and took a seat between a large cube of salt and sugar. Their rough skin was hurtful and some of it brushed against the skin of Miss Lady Leek. "Wow, they are so rough. They need a serious skin exfoliation." She winced in pain. "Probably mixed with me!" Lemon pointed towards himself "Sugar is an excellent exfoliator when mixed with my puss." Lemon gloated.

"She said they need an exfoliation. Not that they are an exfoliator." Mrs Lady Finger rolled her eyes.

"You love praising yourself, don't you?" Miss Lady Leek teased Lemon to which lemon just smiled.

"But right now, stay away from me. Your puss is leaking again," chubby Cauliflower ordered Lemon agitated.

"And the puss is burning my skin and stringing my eyes," Mrs Lady Finger scowled with blur tears in her eyes, formed by the burn from the string of the puss.

"They leak when I am nervous. And I am really nervous about the whole brain thing right now," Lemon cried back.

"And you call yourself a protector. Go and be nervous somewhere else; your puss is too acidic." chubby Cauliflower scowled too offering his handkerchief to Mrs Ladyfinger.

"Where should I go? We are all packed like fishes in this train compartment." Lemon huffed "And you call yourself a protector. Most of your army is stale, not even that fresh like us. You are so inferior to me," he made a face at chubby Cauliflower.

"And it's already stinky over here," Miss Lady Leek exasperated trying to fan the air near her nose with her fingers; in hopes that it would clear the stink.

"That's not because of my puss. It's because of all the blue blood over there," Lemon cried.

"That's true." Other vegetables nodded as they witnessed the blue bloods bubbles flowing in their seats. But thankfully the blue bloods were quite at a distance from their seat; almost at the opposite side of the train.

"Impure blood," Nerdy Spinach Leaf cursed under his breath, seeing those bloods flowing on the opposite side of the train.

A huge led screen in train chamber flashed the train itinerary for the day. A beautiful voice soothed out of it. "Next station: kidney. Blood filtration. Salt and sugar are to be removed. Next station: kidney."

The blue blood bubbles got up from their place and started flowing in their direction. All the vegetables moved back in their seat in fright. Thankfully, they had just passed them without touching them. There were fables that they heard about how a blue blood would impure and damage anything they would touch.

Even the cubes of sugar and salt got up from their seat and moved towards the exit door.

As soon as Kidney station came all three of them got down.

"Next stop: Skin layer. Fibrin for repairing a cut on the skin near the waist. Next stop: Skin Layer." The sing-song voice from LCD Sang again.

Inside the train chamber there were two rows with opposite couches. A family of vitamin B which looked like strips of some paper stood at the entrance door. The vegetable shifted and made some space for them to sit.

"That's very kind of you. Thank you very much," Mrs Vitamin B said politely.

"You are welcome," Miss Lady Leek smiled back.

"We are just bit amused to see vegetables in carbon-dioxide train. By the way, we are vitamin B. But you can also call us B." The female vitamin B said. The vegetables were confused as to from where her sound was coming, since nothing like mouth was moving on her face.

"Yes, we were scared to come in carbon-dioxide train. We thought we would have monstrous experience but nothing of that sort has really happened yet. So far it has been easy." Mrs Lady Finger said relieved and then she continued, "We were so scared we will have to encounter carbon-dioxide."

"Yeah, they have not yet climbed in yet. They will climb at the next stop." The male vitamin B joined in the conversation casually. Even he spoke without any visible mouth moving on his face.

The vegetables shivered hearing that.

"Don't worry they are not that monstrous. They are pretty harmless!" The vitamin B family laughed. "The whole rumour of carbon dioxide being deadly is a fable of somebody's imagination. They are just very irritating," Mrs B rolled her eyes.

"Just like how the breads are going to rule everybody's body one day," chubby Cauliflower laughed along with them.

All the members of vitamin B stopped laughing and turned serious.

"Oh! You very much believe it!" Chubby Cauliflower immediately stopped laughing.

"Yes. Breads are a grave danger to the body, don't you think?" The baby vitamin B asked quietly

"No, I think it's a great fictional horror story." Chubby Cauliflower argued.

A thin Band-Aid got up from opposite couch and proceeded towards door.

"Bye fibrin. Take care," the vitamin B family bid the thin Band-aid a goodbye.

"He repairs skin," mother vitamin B whispered to Mrs Ladyfinger.

Mrs Lady Finger nodded in understanding.

The train came to a stop on a station. They could clearly see a sign post of Skin layer was written over it. Fibrin got down and the train moved again.

"Next station: Pancreas, Vitamin B, a glass of water. Next station: Pancreas." The voice from LCD started speaking again.

"That's our stop. I wish you all best for your journey." Mother Vitamin B hugged Mrs Ladyfinger and Miss Lady Leek. The vitamin B family bid goodbye to the entire troop of vegetables and walked towards the door. Bouncy water molecules followed them behind. A cool sensation passed across the vegetables body as the transparent water molecules passed them.

Once again the train came to a stop on pancreas station, which was hardly at any distance from Skin station.

The temperature of chambers increased. Grey molecules of carbon dioxide bounced towards the opposite side of the couch. They were extremely hot and their heat could be felt by vegetables too. Some of them even started sweating.

Right behind them a female, 'half red-half blue' barrier stepped inside the chamber with her minions following her behind.

The train moved again. And the voice from LED sang again, "Next station Heart. Next station: heart."

"Listen everyone," The two-coloured barrier spoke. "Somebody has exchanged their cards with the family of B-amino acids. They are panicked and have moist eyes. Kindly give them their cards back or be prepared to be thrown in toilet jail for theft." Blood barrier roared evilly with a determined glint in her eyes. Her red colour kept fading to blue as the minute went by. It was very creepy, actually to be honest.

"Check everyone's bag." She ordered her team. Her minions started opening bags one by one. "This has never happened in the circulatory system before. You know why?" She looked at everyone, "Because we are not like that pathetic digestive system. We are known to never fail or get upset like a stomach, because we are organised and systematic. We do everything perfectly. Nobody can just hop and take this train for a ride." She ranted on top of her voice as she inspected everyone's faces thoroughly.

All the vegetables shifted lower in their seats scared. They pulled out their cards and rightly so, the words "amino acid" was written right there on it. Chubby Cauliflower tightened his hands nervously.

"Oh my god! We are doomed. We are all going to die in the toilet jail," Miss Lady Leek exclaimed horrified.

"I say, we act normally and get down at Heart station before they see us," Chubby Cauliflower whispered to Spinach Leaf.

"Right in front of their eyes" Spinach Leaf retorted sarcastically. "You don't really think it through before opening your mouth now, do you? You genius!"

"So do you have a better plan?" Chubby Cauliflower whispered back harshly.

The minions were all throwing open the bags and spewing contents of it on ground while barrier kept at a vigilant glare on them. They rummaged through the bags and double-checked each document.

"I see. You are being smart and alert. But it will be only before time, when I snatch you by your collar and drag you to toilet jail by myself," Barrier squeaked to no-one in particular clenching and unclenching her fist.

One of the minions moved forward and stood in front of Miss Lady Leek. Miss Lady Leek jumped and gave out a sharp cry.

"I am sorry, didn't see you there," Miss Lady Leek apologised, clenching her heart tightly.

"AHHHH. See who we have here 'the protectors'!" barrier squeaked evilly as she sized them up from toe-to-head. She walked towards them slowly. "Protectors of intestine feels they can roam anywhere in the body, wherever they please, without a ticket, breaking the rules, stealing and committing theft, putting the whole body in grave danger. Taking the body for granted. Thinking that I am a fool! Thinking that whole circulatory system is fool! Committing a crime and sitting there like nothing has happened," Barrier went in loud rant again. She inched her face closer to chubby Cauliflower till there were only a few centimetres between their faces, "But I am not a fool. You are a fool to think I am fool. I will prison you in toilet jail and they will churn and churn out all your juices till the time you are nothing but urine. Then you know what happens to the urine. Don't you?" Barrier cooed while chubby cauliflower nodded his head frantically, sweat beading on his forehead.

"Goodbye from the body!" She ended with her signature evil smirk, showing just a tooth.

"Found it," the minions declared, after searching an overhead shelve. They too were losing their red colour quicker and becoming bluer than before.

Barrier huffed annoyed at her minion. All vegetables let out the relief sighs they were holding in.

She looked at her minion with annoyance. She huffed and backed away from the vegetables with a sour face; she snatched the card from her minion's hands. There was a positive amino B written right on the top of it.

Chapter 9

Heart

Next station: - Right heart:- for a push to the lungs at a quick speed. Fasten your seatbelts. I repeat Fasten your seatbelt. Next station:- Right heart."

"I didn't understand a word. Push where?" Mrs Lady Finger wined.

"Don't let spinach hear that," chubby Cauliflower laughed.

"It's too complicated," Mrs Lady Finger whispered back confused.

"Fasten your seat belt quick. We are in for a long Push," Nerdy Spinach Leaf whispered hurriedly to both of them.

As the train entered the right heart, blood gushed towards it at a top speed. The entire train was now floating on the blood. It pushed and carried forward the train with full gusto. Soon the blood enveloped the train from all the sides. The train which was once floating over the red blood was now swimming in middle of that very blood.

It was like the train was in middle of a blood storm, being rattled and rustled along with the gushing flow of the blood. The train was swirling in circles like a cloth in the washing machine.

After being pushed forward ferociously, they were now being pushed backwards, before being pushed forward again with a new force; back and forth it went on for some-time. Their train was now being pushed to another chamber of heart through a narrow tube. The vegetables were being thrown off their seats and fell down from their couch. They were pushed from one end of the train to another due to lack of balance. Lemon was hit on his head. Puss started oozing out from it. Mrs Lady Finger too lost her balance, but chubby Cauliflower caught her in his arms. Miss Lady Leek tried to push down her skirt which had climbed up her thighs. While Bitter-Gourd held on to one of the poles tightly, Garden Peas were busy swinging from one end of the train to another. It was an absolute madness with nobody able to keep up with their balance.

The train was now in the second right chamber of the heart. Like the first chamber, in second chamber too their train was again floating like a fish in the middle of the blood. It rushed downwards towards the bottom of the second right chamber steadily for a few seconds.

But then their train again climbed upwards and in mild mini seconds they were sucked in another tube at a high speed. They were drifting in that tube at an abnormally high speed. Soon they were pushed from that tube too. All the vegetables screamed as the train shook violently and their heads bashed against the walls.

Their hair was flying in all directions. They were screaming at the top of their lungs, trying to make sense of what was happening. It was a hurricane and they were right in the middle of it. Chubby Cauliflower did not let go of Lady Finger's hand, even for a second which she was grateful for. Miss Lady Leek had her eyes closed and jaws clenched. Lemon did not know how to control his puss from leaking. His puss was now dropped all over the train floor. Wise Bitter-Gourd was keeping calm. While all the peas were now thrown out of their pod.

Even through all this madness the voice from LCD sang again and it was as smooth as butter.

Next station:- lungs: Carbon dioxide for exhale, Oxygen for filtration. Next station: - lungs.

"Can't she catch a break even in this blood storm?" Lemon questioned the voice from T.V unbelievingly.

Finally the train calmed down. And the storm died. It was now floating in the air like an aeroplane in the sky. And all the vegetables got up from their floor and took their seats like how the passengers of a turbulent airplane in movies would after the weather calms down. They could see white conical strips below them through the window.

The grey bubbles which had occupied half of the chamber stood up. Along with them, many oxygen bubbles stuck with dust particles to them stood up which almost emptied the entire train. Those oxygen bubbles looked tired by all the weight of dust particles stuck to them.

"They look like they could use a good bath!" Miss Lady Leek gossiped to Mrs. Lady Finger. "Oh wait! They are going to the lungs for a nice makeover. They will be purified by the cleansing ladies in the lungs. Then they will look their glowing and beautiful red again."

While all the bubbles stood elegantly at the door, the vegetables were still trying hard to keep their balance in their seats. Outside their window they could witness white conical stripes below. Inside that white stripes were a grey coloured station.

They were now floating between the gushy winds, before the train again found its track as they approached the oncoming station from a distance. The board at station spelled lung station. They were finally in lungs. They could feel the fresh air of lungs coming in the chambers of train. The vegetables could finally breathe the fresh air again.

They also heaved a sigh of relief when they saw a now-total blue blood barrier, distracted by screaming and shouting at her minions.

They looked at their cards again and saw just "amino acid" was written on it and not B-amino acid, like what the blood barrier was finding for a minute ago. This time they were saved by the bell, But that was short lived, as they could again see, the now-dark-blue blood barrier looking at them intensely. Smoke was vaporising out of her nose. She walked towards them like a blue cat. She halted in front of them. "Show me your tickets." She purred, like a cat.

Now it was turn for vegetables to lose all the colour of their face and turn blue. They gulped and then gulped some more. With shaking hands, they handed over the tickets to her.

"I knew it," She fisted her hand victoriously in air when she saw their cards. "You all are just a bunch of thieves, protectors my foot!" She screamed. All her minions came forward towards them with an evil smirk on their face. They caught the collars of vegetables and kicked them outside the train. The vegetables landed on the ground of station with oomph.

The station was sophisticatedly built and fully oxygenated. The station had grey bony interior and it was all trapped in white conical stripes. They all knew it was Ribs as soon as they saw white conical stripes up in the sky. The ceiling of the station was also constantly falling in and out from constant inhalation and exhalations. Though there was warmth and moist in the air, the wind was thick and gushing. There were some big and small cyclones and storms happening at some places on the station. The ambience was pleasant nevertheless. Bitter Gourd almost felt like he was back in Himalayas. He always talked about how he swayed on the hills. Now everybody was swaying in winds along with him.

They saw heavy winds blowing in their direction. It scared Mrs. Lady Finger.

"My parents used to protect me in storms and rains fearing that I would get infected. I find them terrifying!" Mrs Lady Finger cried.

"Don't worry. It's not going to rain over here, just the winds blowing heavily," chubby Cauliflower soothed her.

"But why are there so many winds over here?" Mrs. Lady Finger sobbed.

"It's lungs! It's filled with air," Lemon told her unbelievably.

"But don't get sucked in those winds. You will be never found again," wise Bitter-Gourd warned.

They got up from the place they had fallen down to avoid getting sucked in the winds blowing in their direction.

At their right was a cleaning shop. Billions of tiny hair strands were standing at its entrance. They were busy shouting trying to get vegetables' attention.

"Sir, do you want to get cleaned? We will clean you in half the price of the other cleaning shop in the Lung station." All the hair spoke together in their rough hairy voice. One might wonder what a hairy voice might be!

"Okay! But we don't have a rupee," the wise-Bitter Gourd complained.

"Fine then, we will do it for free," they all chorused together again. All the rough voice chorusing together was definitely very irritating to their ears.

They all started walking towards the shop. Whenever ceiling of station caved in, they bent down on the floor and they got up again as soon as the ceiling caved out. They entered the shop. Its interiors were hair-themed. Walls were decorated with tiny hair. Those tiny hairs were differently styled at different places. Some had knot patterns on them. Some other where, it was combed and knot-free. While some patch were pretending to be braided. Other patch pretended to be French bun. Somewhere they were tied up in pony, some other-where they were left open.

'Real cleansing job.' 'Real cleansing job.' Slogan adorned on walls at various patches in the shop.

"I wonder who the owner is!" Miss Lady Leek wondered in amazement.

“I am.” A rough voice spoke, as a bit taller than other hair strands, but still not even reaching an inch hair-strand presented itself from behind a table.

“I am Cillia. And I run this shop,” his voice was extremely rough and dry. It needed some serious conditioning.

“Stand in the line, please, if you want to get cleaned,” He gestured them towards a line.

All the vegetables stood in a huge Line. Ahead of them were those very same off- red coloured bubbles from the train, who looked exhausted by having dust particles sticking to them. They were dirty as if rolled in dust and their red colour lacked lustre and passion. Miss Lady Leek nudged Mrs Lady Finger to remind her they were the same people they were gossiping about.

There was a belt right in front of the line. All the billion hair particles, who were initially pleading them to enter the shop, had now inserted themselves in the patch of the belt. They waved back and forth in the gushing winds of lungs like a crop in the wind. The first red bubble in line dragged its feet in front of those hairs. Immediately the billions of hair stopped swaying. They became paralysed. The few millions in the billions started sneezing then. “This bubble is just too contaminated,” one of the hair said. The billion of hair again resumed their movement. They were cleaning the bubble of the dust stuck on it. They were also trying to purify the air around it.

“And it has a lot of contaminated air around it,” the other who was still not moving and continuously sneezing said.

“Yes loads of it,” the third one sneezed and resumed back its work of cleaning the blood molecule like others.

The red blood bubble was shiny and sparkly again. Cillia thanked the bubble for choosing their services.

“Thank you for using our services.” All the billion hair particle also appreciated the bubble together.

One by one, other bubbles in line moved towards the belt and placed their feet in front of the hair particles. They started sapping all their dirt. But the dust of the bubbles was too high for the hair to bear. Most of them started dying. Few of them started choking. “This is the tenth time dust is blowing on me.” A hair particle choked. His throat is extremely dry. "One more time, and I am going to die." And he dies when the dust blew on him again.

"Ohh" they all screamed horrified, "one more dies because of dust."

Other hair particles also started choking and holding their neck, "We are going to die if this dust is continuously blown on us."

"Cut the drama." Cillia screamed at them as vegetables looked at the hair strands tucked in belt weirdly. Next was their turn and they were disgusted having to stand in front of thousands of hair.

"Don't worry! They will make you sparkly again." Cillia spoke to vegetables to encourage them to step in front of the belt.

Lemon was the first one to step in front of the hair. The hair stated wiggling on his body, making him feel ticklish. He used to constantly roll-off from in front of them making it difficult for hair strands to clean him. Also, most of them started screaming when his puss started leaking on the floor.

"This is horrible. This creature doesn't know how to stand properly in front of us." One of the hair strand complained to cilia.

"Yes! It's very difficult. He doesn't have feet to stand." Another wined.

"And his puss is leaking from his body. It's dirtying the floor." They all complained.

After his cleaning was finally done, they all heaved a sigh of relief. And thanked God he was gone from front of their eyes.

After him, Miss Lady Leek stepped in front of them. The hair strands started cleaning her entire body at once.

"No don't! Don't, please. This is too rough for my delicate skin." She screamed when thousands of hair strands started rubbing against her body.

"No don't you dare touch me like that." She screamed at one strand when he lifted her skirt a bit to clean it there.

"O woman! How else am I supposed to clean you?" The hair strand questioned her. When she was finally done, she swore it was a nightmare.

Mrs Lady Finger and chubby Cauliflower decided to make their relationship finally official and stepped in front of the belt together. "Aww" the hair particles crooned at them when they saw them hand-in-hand. They started giggling as the hair particles started cleaning them together. "You guys look lovely together." one hair particle complimented them while other said he would have taken their picture if she had a camera. After a lot of "aww" and "ahh" they were finally done.

When Bitter-Gourd stepped in front of hair, they all placed their hands on their nose. His bitter smell was repellent and they quickly finished off his cleaning. Nerdy Spinach Leaf refused to get cleaned by the hair, even though they pleaded him, fearing they would break his glasses. Garden peas were the last, who bounced happily in front of hair. Immediately the hair started cleaning it on all its curves.

After a certain minute, they exited the shop all shining and sparkling except Nerdy Spinach Leaf who was still the same.

They all walked towards the staircase at the end of the platform. They climbed the grey stairs made of bones.

There was a small gas shop in the corner of the stairs. There was a huge line of blue blood bubbles in front of shop. They were the same blue bubbles from the train. They all looked depressed and lacked energy. They were waiting for their turn to enter the shop.

At the top of the bony stairs, there was a grey bony corridor.

A transparent and glowing neon-yellow- looking- potato- shaped-creature was standing in corridor with his mouth wide open. His eyes and ears were alerted as soon he saw a fly flying too close to him. "Must have come with mouth while yawning." He wondered in his head. Suddenly he wrapped himself around the body of the fly, saw him in the eye, opened his mouth wide and gulped it at once. He licked his mouth after a burp. "I hate trespassers." He roared.

All the vegetables stood there stunned. To shocked to move. They had just witnessed a murder of fly at the hands of a neon glowing Potato.

Garden peas got excited and started waving at him while others asked to shush it down and not to attack his attention.

"Shush!" Nerdy Spinach Leaf said irritated.

"That's our old friend potato." The peas gushed excited.

"Calm down girls! That not potato...That's phagocyte." Wise Bitter-Gourd tried to calm their excitement.

"Maybe after he sacrificed, he got posted over here." Garden Pea suggested.

"I am pretty sure that's not how it works." Wise Bitter Gourd voiced doubtfully. "That's phagocyte. He eats trespassers."

"Well we are not trespassers." Peas said hurt. "We are protectors."

"In lungs we are trespassers," Nerdy Spinach Leaf argued.

"It is a potato! Even this is yellow coloured. So what, it's transparent. It doesn't make it any less potato. This is absurd", the peas argued back. "Potato" they screamed at him.

The phagocyte looked up from his position and smiled back at the smiling peas.

"See I told you he is potato." They bounced excitedly. They all took a step towards him to hug him.

But before they knew and could walk further the phagocyte had crossed all the distance and in blink of eye, wrapped himself around the chubby Cauliflower.

He saw chubby Cauliflower in eye. He saw his terrified, full of fear eyes and took a bite of his body.

"O Lord!" All the other vegetable screamed.

"Murder!" chubby Cauliflower yelled.

"Trespasser!" He yelled back at them.

"We are not trespassers." Peas yelled back. "Mind your tongue." Phagocyte ignored it and opened his mouth wide again for another bite of Cauliflower.

The chubby Cauliflower cried in pain but he still couldn't move since he was still stuck in his clutch.

"Leave him." They all tried to separate the phagocyte from the Cauliflower. But he was stuck to him like glue. He again opened his mouth and was about to take a bite when Spinach Leaf finally pulled him and unglued him from his body.

Bitter-Gourd had caught a nearby passing fly and threw it in a distance, when phagocyte was looking. He immediately ran to catch it. He wrapped himself against the fly and gulped it down in one bite. It freaked out the vegetables.

"Let's go before he comes back for us." Nerdy Spinach Leaf suggested and they all ran towards the stairs they had come from. The phagocyte ran behind them, but stopped after a while.

"I watch this lobby. Do not come back. Ever!" he shouted at them from the back as they climbed down the bony stairs.

It wasn't helping either that in between of their run, the ceiling was continuously caving in on them and they had to duck down after every few seconds.

They saw an oxygen train pulling up to the lung station. A voice on a speaker announced its arrival.

As soon as they saw the phagocyte climbing down the stairs and coming behind them all vegetable protectors swiped their amino cards into the train slot and then jumped into the train.

They pushed open the doors and walked inside. A small round red particle made an irritated face when he saw them entering.

Chapter 10

Push!!!!

"We don't have space for too many? Please few of you get down?" The particle said in an irritated voice.

"No we need everybody, as we have to fight bread, save beetroots and bring them back." Nerdy Spinach Leaf told the particle straight and determined. He was now tired from all the running.

The train was jam-packed full but it was true that they had to reach the brain to release beetroots and bring them back.

"Huh! I see! Again captured." Particle spoke with wide eyes. Then he looked at his fellow nutrients in the train. "Guys rearrange yourself, and make space for our guest."

All the white blood cells and red blood cells in train twisted themselves into some odd shape to make space for all the vegetables. Vegetables went and sat beside them.

"I am a tidy housekeeper and do not like anything cluttering up my premises." A jolly voice boomed from the other side of the train. All vegetables turned their head towards the voice. It was another red coloured barrier. This Barrier had a nice smile on her face. They all panicked as she was coming in their direction. They immediately rushed in the corner and hide behind a pillar. Two nutrients were standing right in front of them.

"Let me inform you about our itinerary. We will go straight to brain but after a push from heart. Hope we have a good push," Barrier announced happily to all the passengers in train.

"Yay!!!" everybody clapped at the word "good" and vegetables sighed at the name of heart. Heart was violent.

"Alright! I guess." Mrs Lady Finger said exhausted, just hearing about it. "Let's do it." She added in faint quiet voice.

"I hope we get a good pump from heart today!" The nutrient in front of them was discussing it with the other nutrient in front of them.

"It's been years now since the train was directly pumped to the brain," the other nutrient nodded along.

"Those were some golden years," the first one sighed.

The Particle came looking for vegetables.

"Where did you all go? We got so worried," he told them disappointedly.

The vegetables sighed and walked back to their earlier seats along with the particle.

While moving, Miss Lady Leek's hand brushed against the nutrient ahead unintentionally. "Sorry," she apologised to the nutrient.

"No problem." She smiled at her.

On their seat all the cells were curious and gathered around the protectors to ask them questions.

"Have you ever been to brain before?" One of them asked with loads of interest.

"Not without digestion." Wise Bitter-Gourd replied.

"Wow. Then that's like you guys are making some history. Like first vegetables to land on the brain without digestion like the first man to land on moon," the cells said in amazement. "Blimey! Do you have a flag to go along with this?"

"Blimey no." Nerdy Spinach Leaf said bitterly, "We need to concentrate on finding beetroots!"

Now the Barrier was checking everyone's cards few paces from them. She was happily chatting with a bunch of glucoses.

"Did you check the bread spread in the blood?" A passenger Glucose asked blood barrier.

"What a mess," the blood barrier agreed.

"Yes! Spreading as if vacationing on a beach!" The passenger Glucose said disgusted.

The vegetables slid a little lower in their places wishing the bottom of the train would just gulp them up. Besides them the cells were busy discussing their own thing.

"I don't know what she is thinking?" One of the cell wondered.

"Not eating whole day is horrible too. Then suddenly eating at night like a crazy woman! " The first cell added.

Vegetables sighed. Seemed like heart pump and body was hot topic in the oxygen train. Everybody was discussing it. The train had left the grey lung organ and they were going to heart for a good push.

****

Tee's night sleep starts with a terrifying dream of not just a big but an extremely big girl stuck in a manhole. The whole school which had circled her were laughing on her mercilessly. Her mum begged and pleaded them not to laugh at her. She was continuously trying to get out of the hole but she was stuck. The whole school was howling and roaring. "Please don't laugh at her!" her mother begged, "Please! So what if she is fat? So what if doctor said it will take her 36 surgeries to remove the fat?" those words of mum cracked their laughs some more and now they were practically chuckling more loudly while some rolling on earth with delight. Her mum pleaded them to shush down and not hurt her feelings. Her crush Jay passed by the hole, paused for a moment, took pity on her and then started walking again. His arms were slung around her friend j's waist, who had an "I- told-you-so-face."

She woke up from her dream with a start. Sweat beading on her forehead. A sharp pain coursed through tee's heart. Her heart was racing now. She could feel all her muscles contracting themselves, piling one beat over another. She took a deep breath in and out. Listen to some soulful music. She could feel her muscles releasing its tension and slowly relaxing themselves again.

Soon her dream of people laughing on her was replaced by cheese grilled double-decker sandwich with soda as drink, which calmed her heart and she went back to sleep peacefully.

****

The train had just entered the left side of heart. And was once again was floating between the blood.

"How romantic! We are in heart" chubby Cauliflower whispered in Miss Lady Finger's ears while she blushed.

"My love!" he whispered back under his breath.

"Don't worry! As soon as the heart gets stormy it won't be that romantic." Nerdy Spinach Leaf spoke with a straight face staring at the couple.

Chubby Cauliflower stared at him for ruining their moment. Spinach gave him a fake smile in return.

"OMG! We are doomed. She is coming right here." Miss Lady Leek exclaimed.

And true to her words the barrier was coming right at them to check their cards. She had a jovial smile on her face. But suddenly at that moment the train started shaking violently and she tripped and fell down. Along with her many nutrients fell from their seat, piling up on one above the other. Another violent jerk and everybody started screaming. Everybody grabbed on to the poles, bones, muscles and whatever they could hold on to for the support. Muscles of heart had started contracting. The whole train was pushed backwards. The blood around the train was getting torrential. It was swimming around them ferociously. The whole oxygen train was shaking and swinging violently. There was turbulence in heart.

"The girl is having a nightmare!" The cell from besides concluded.

"Again?" The other cell asked surprised.

Yes. It's happening quite every night from a month." The third cell said irked, "Why does this girl always have to be on fire in her dreams?"

"That's what a nightmare is called." The first cell rolled his eyes sarcastically.

"Now all that panicking is again going to leave a scar in the heart. The scar looks like an ugly pea." The second cell shook her head disappointingly.

All the peas in pod looked angrily towards him.

"And she is so dull in the day, and jumpy in night. It's confusing the body." The cell continued speaking ignoring the peas.

"We just got a message from the brain. The Heart is in the full panicky mode." The Barrier spoke concerned her hands on her chest.

"Now this heart is going to race itself to death." The passenger glucose declared.

"Don't worry help will be here. The brain has signalled nose to take deeper breaths and Ears to listen to soulful music for meditation." Barrier tried to pacify everyone.

"It surely needs to relax. When the chica worries, the heart worries! When the chica calms, the heart calms down!" The first cell spoke scared.

"She is worsening everything due to her unnecessary worrying." Glucose nodded his head disappointedly.

All the muscles which had contracted themselves were now relaxing themselves back. They could feel the heart calm down. All of them heaved a sigh of relief.

"Mission successful! The girl is calm again and the brain did it again. Or else I honestly felt the girl wouldn't survive another night." One of the cells spoke.

"Exactly! It's miraculous!" The other cells agreed.

"Hopefully the heart will push nicely now."

"Yes last time it only pushed till shoulders. It was such a weak push."

All the cells started discussing amongst themselves. They had a long climb to the brain and a big push by heart was desired from quite some months now.

The heart soon started preparing itself for a big push. What started slowly and calmly was now gushing in the middle of the heart.

A long tube was present in the middle of the heart .The train was now slowly getting sucked towards that long tube at a rapid speed. Within a fraction of a second, the train was inside the tube. Then it went on and on ahead inside the tube.

"Push!" they all screamed encouragingly together inside the train.

Everything was happening in a 'blink of eye' speed. In the tube, there were a few pushes back and forth before they were pumped outside the tube with a roaring speed. Everything went rushing behind as they went upwards at a lightning speed. It was a complete blur when the vegetables tried looking from the window.

But sadly the vehicle soon started losing its momentum. The vehicle which was at full speed was now slowly coming to a halt. It finally came to a stop and landed on a thin bone. The whole vehicle was now hanging upside down on that thin bone.

Her peaceful sleep was short lived as her throat started hiccupping without a warning. Her throat felt heavy and her hiccups were quite strong. She went to the kitchen and drank down a glass of water. She waited for hiccups to die, but they were now stronger than ever. She drank another glass of water, but even after that she felt she might have to drink a few more glasses. So she now drowned down a bottle. Finally, she gave up and went back to bed still hiccupping.

The train got stuck on bone and was constantly threatening to fall down from it.

All the vegetables fell down from their seat. The cells helped the vegetables to get up, but they themselves fell down when the bone in the throat on which the train hanged started hiccupping. The bone started shaking and making sounds. It was making the position of train on the bone even more vulnerable. The train was ready to fall down at any moment. Whenever the bone shook the whole train would shake along with it. Once again everybody inside the train grabbed on to the poles, bones, muscles and whatever they could find to maintain their balance. To add to their troubles, soon they were drowned down with water. All of them got wet inside the train. The pressure of water loosened the grip of the train over the bone more. Soon enough more and more water started pouring over and inside the train. The vegetables were drenched along with all the other nutrients in train. The bone started hiccupping more powerfully than ever before and the train started shaking violently over the bone. Everybody inside the train started shivering from the cold water. Finally the water stopped pouring and the train stopped shaking. Even the hiccups died and the train could start climbing itself up again.

All of them let out a sigh of relief. "We are fine." The nutrients spoke composed as they climbed up from where they had fallen down. "All is fine."

The train was now slowly climbing up the side of the face. The insides of the face were steep and sharp. It was a bony maze with bones coming out from everywhere. The face was extremely narrow and hardly had any cheeks.

"Wow! It's so bony! I can only see bones and bones everywhere." Miss Lady Leek exclaimed.

"No I can see her room too!' Nerdy Spinach Leaf spoke as he went near the window and looked out of it. They all followed him near the window and stared outside world in amazement.

They could all see her lovely room through her slightly opened lips.

The girl had moist and pouted lips. There was a tub of saliva dripping outside her lips. They could also see the up and down erect pillars of teeth. The teeth were biting her lips slightly.

"Aww!" They all gaped in amazement as they felt the wind blow on their face. They could feel the wind coming in through the slightly opened mouth.

"It's such a beautiful night!" Chubby Cauliflower said, looking in Mrs Lady Finger's eyes.

"A true joy ride!" Mrs Lady Finger answered back looking in his eyes.

"Then where are the stars? There are stars at night." Lemon wondered aloud.

"She is in her room, you doofus!" Nerdy Spinach Leaf scolded him.

"Ticket please!" The red Barrier came and stood beside them. There was kindness in her eyes and a smile on her lips. Seeing her standing beside them, the vegetables started shivering in their pants. They looked at each other in panic. In all the excitement, they had completely forgotten about her.

"Delightful, isn't it? That's why I like my job. I get to travel a lot. Yesterday I had a delivery to make in foot area. I got to explore the majestic legs and thighs." She started up a conversation with them happily.

"Of course! I went to other areas too." She giggled. "You know what areas I am talking about right?" She asked blushingly. She was now red. She was already very red. But now her cheeks were redder than ever.

All the vegetables were literally shivering now. They nodded at whatever she was saying, but beneath the façade they were shivering and sweating.

"That was good pump by heart, aye?" She asked them still happily.

"Aye." they all nodded in agreement. Sweat dripping down their face.

"Well not that good. We were stuck on the throat bone and were going to fall down but we managed to overcome it nevertheless. It's been ages since the heart pushed the train straight to the brain." She sighed. "You know what this means, right?" she asked them.

They all shaked their head from one side to another which meant a 'no.'

"This means we will have to climb all the way up through the face. It's going to be difficult through all this bones." She informed them.

"But it's picturesque. So it won't be that bad. In fact it would be delightful." She added delightfully.

All the vegetables pretended to nod along with whatever she said.

"It's funny to see the protectors in the train. I have never seen any protector before in train." She told them confused, "It's a pleasant surprise though. But I hope you have the ticket?" She asked them sweetly.

"Of course we do!" Lemon spoke quickly.

"Yes! Of course we do. We wouldn't enter without it. Nobody can. This is not digestive route." They all laughed it off nervously as the biggest joke of century.

All the nutrients and Barrier were staring at vegetables expectantly to show up their ticket. Barrier even raised her eyebrow in expectation. The vegetables had no luck but to put their hand inside their pocket and bring out the tickets of amino acids. They handed it over to the barrier with shaky hands.

After checking the card on both the sides thoroughly she looked at them sternly.

"Your own I meant! This is of amino family." She told them in a calm voice

"VV..W..We don't ha-have our own." They told her in a stuttering voice.

"Thought so when you all started laughing unnecessarily." She told them surprising in a kind and calm tone.

"You know how ridiculously risky it is for unregistered particles to enter the heart? We all could have been killed. The girl could have been killed." She explained to them sweetly. "And it's my job to make sure that no unregistered particle enters the heart. It would have been my fault."

The Vegetables did not speak a word and stood there silently in front of her.

"What could possibly make a protector endanger the body?" She asked them with not even a hint of anger in her voice. Like how a therapist would ask his patient a question. She was genuinely trying to understand why the protectors of body, intestine, to be precise would take such a grave step.

"King bread kidnapped beetroots! And we are trying to bring them back." Wise Bitter-Gourd spoke after a few minutes of silence. The cells besides them nodded along. Barrier just stood there trying to take in whatever the wise Bitter-Gourd just said. Her eyes welled up after a while and a tear streamed down her cheek.

"That's so noble!" She clapped, "I am genuinely touched." And then she proceeded to hug everyone.

The vegetables were taken aback by her gesture and looked at each other weirdly before hugging her back.

"Body needs Beetroots to make blood and you are going to the brain to bring them back. No previous protector has ever done such a noble deed for the body." She said wiping her tears. Her nose had turned cherry red and her eyes were full of hopes and determination.

"That's indeed noble." The cells added besides them.

"Promise me you will bring them back!" She looked Bitter Gourd with all the honesty and sincerity. "Because only you protectors can save us now and heal this body." Barrier asked Bitter Gourd with lots of faith.

"We will my friend. We will." He told her determined.

"Be safe." Barrier said and Bitter Gourd nodded as she left them alone and moved on to the next nutrient to check their card.

"She has colour of my then neighbour cherries." Mrs Lady Finger whispered in the ears Miss Lady Leek.

"Thought I am kind and generous, I am also a tidy housekeeper," Barrier said, eyeing the lemon particularly. Lemon immediately wiped the puss he had dropped and smiled foolishly at the blood barrier.

They went back to looking outside the window of the train. The train was now extremely slow and making its way up the sharp cheek bones. Girl's cheeks were sucked in and hardly had any cushioning. Hence it looked more raw and edgy from inside.

They could again see the outside world through the holes of the nose. Mostly they could see the whole body of a girl outside the hole. The beautiful brown skin of face and how her belly rose and fell in sleep! The body was their home. Their beautiful home!

Her lips even looked curvier and redder from the nose hole. It was fascinating. But its view kept obstructing because of heavy wind blowing ferociously in the nose. As if the nose was having a hurricane. It kept sucking in the air heavily through its hole.

The vegetables had even heard about how the humans loved putting their fingers in nose.

"They say there is an ancient treasure buried in nose. The wind keeps blowing there to safeguard the treasure from the thieves."

Nerdy Spinach spoke about the fable he had read from professor's library.

"That's why humans love putting their fingers in nose that much. To dig the treasure!" Mrs Lady Finger concluded.

"Yeah that's why they dig their nose." They all agreed.

Outside window on their right were beautiful carvings of ears. They looked like they were sculpted by a painter. They could once again see the outside world, right through the small holes of the ears. They could see the beautiful curtains of the girl's room and beautiful fairy lights shimmering outside her window.

"Wow!" They all gazed adoringly.

They were now climbing further towards the eyes. The eyes were a bit open and they gawked at the stars and moon pattern in the ceiling of her room. They could even see the eyes being protected by bunch of hair. They were perfectly curved like how a perfect eyelid should be. But they also had white particles sprinkled in it.

"Eww! That's dandruff. Gross." Miss Lady Leek grunted as she saw the white particles.

They were now heading towards the brain and they saw the barrier coming towards the vegetables with panicky eyes. "We will soon approach the brain. As soon as we reach the entrance there will be a river. Get down from the back doors and swim the river."

"What? Why would we do that?" Miss Lady Leek asked alert.

"Because the barriers guarding the brain entrance has been replaced by brown n black bread loaf."

"Ohh!!" They whispered.

"They will inspect the train and if they see you, they will capture and put you in the memory loss jail of the brain." Barrier gushed out her words worried.

"We will have to swim the river to go inside the brain to avoid being inspected by the bread loafs at the entrance." Lemon straightened it out.

The barrier nodded and left them alone again. All of the vegetables looked at each other worried.

As they were approaching the brain, they could see the dream projectors were on. The girl was dreaming about cheese grilled double Decker sandwich with soda as drink.

"Once upon a time, not too long time back, the girl used to dream about guys, going on dates, dressing up like a princess, doing hair n makeup. Things used to be exciting in the brain. There were good feelings. Now it's just a bunch of videos repeated daily about eating bread." Cell told the Vegetables sadly.

Soon they reached the entrance of the brain. There was a huge river besides it. The train came to halt in front its gates.

The Barrier which used to once guard the gate, were now replaced by proud looking brown and white loafs of bread.

"Glucose and nutrients for the brain." The kind barrier of the train announced on their arrival to loafs.

"Magic words please." The white bread asked proudly.

"Hail the kingdom of the king bread. Long live the king bread," the Barrier spoke with a dead-expression.

"Not the long version, but the short version." The white bread shook his head in amusement.

"Love you king bread!" The barrier spoke again. Her blood was boiling now.

"Damn! Where do you get so much glucose from? this human hardly eats anything under the Sun." the brown bread asked shaking his head in amusement.

"From the extra storage! Can we go now?" the barrier asked irked.

"You see the picture up there." The white bread loaf asked, pointing towards the screen of the projector. Currently extra butter was being spread on a white loaf in the projector. "Those are my brothers. Tomorrow the first thing this human will do is eat my brothers. We will be re-united here man. Here." The white bread hooted and shouted.

"Where man, where?" Bread motioned with hand for barrier to speak up.

"Here."

"Where?"

"Here."

"Where?"

"Here."

"Hey, can we go now? The king might really require the blood and glucose." Barrier said fuming with fury now.

"First let me check whether your train is not carrying any toxic substance to poison our king with." The brown bread suggested, mimicking to check the train.

"Alright. I guess." Barrier said with a chill daunting on her face.

"Roar! I am just kidding Woman." The brown bread said roaring with laughter. "White! Did you see her face?"

"Hey man! Don't call me white. It's racist!" White bread shook his head.

"But on the other hand." Brown bread said poker-faced. "I will check the train. What's in the train?" He asked as he climbed on the train.

"Nutrients 50%"

"White and red cells 49%" Sweat started forming on the forehead of Barrier whiles he spoke. The bread passed him and checked each chamber of train thoroughly.

"Glucose level 25%"

"You may go. You are holding up a line." The brown bread told to barrier after he was satisfied with his inspection.

The Barrier heaved a sigh of relief. At a distance she saw the vegetables swimming in the river and reaching the doors of the brain.

Tee logged in her Facebook account. Her wall was filled with notifications. Mostly they were of J! J gone to a couture show in Paris! J was eating a French cheese Toast in front of the Eiffel tower! J's hair blowing in the wind! J Flirting with a French man called Pierre! J swimming in the river! J blah and J blah! But what caught her eyes was that Jay had liked all her pictures. A pang of jealously hit Tee. He had never liked any of her pictures. Granted, they had never talked to each other in months, but still it hurt her. Though she had to admit J looked quite charming in all her pictures. Her white sun glasses looked stylish on her face and her Dress fitted her like a dream. Her hair left open, flew in the wind and she was pouting in almost all the pictures.

Tee felt sad and a deep hurt ran through her. If only she was as thin as J, she would have had carried those dresses with as much grace as she did. But Alas! She wasn't and nothing was working for her.

Last Week J had shown her a trick which she said was magical for all times she over- ate. It was early morning and they were in their school bathroom to check their hair in the mirror. Tee was still feeling incredibly guilty about eating so much from previous night. She was almost on verge of crying. J sighed and asked Tee to look carefully as she placed her two fingers deep in her own mouth. For few seconds nothing happened but after a moment she started vomiting all the food she had for breakfast.

Tee looked at her vomit in a shock. For a moment she was taken aback. J still continued to vomit. After she was done she washed her mouth with water and wiped her lips. She smiled at her. Tee Looked back at her shocked.

"Now you do it!" J coaxed, asking Tee to repeat her actions.

Tee shook her head scared. She wouldn't do it. The sight of J doing it was too frightening.

"Common! You want to be thin right." J Sighed irritated, "Everybody over-eats sometimes. It's Okay. Just vomit it out." She encouraged her to vomit just like her. Thankfully bell rang, and Tee was saved. She quickly excused herself and rushed out of the bathroom.

That sight still gave her shivers whenever she thought about it. Did Jay know about all the stuff J would do to remain thin? Would he like her pictures then? She had even noticed both of them flirting sometimes. J had always liked him. If only guys knew about the length a girl went to impress them.

She went through other people's pictures. There was her old school teacher playing with her white cat which Tee had gifted her. Her brother was still abroad and her extended family was having a pool party.

While she was glancing through everybody's pictures something at side caught her eyes, "Lose weight in a week", read the heading. A glossy picture of a bottle with a tin cap flashed besides it. "7 kg's gone in 7 days." Tee read out the paragraph described on the Tin bottle loud. "Order our hunger suppressant pills immediately to become extremely thin. Cost of shipping is free."

Tee smiled. A gleam of hope broke through her heart. Was this her final chance to become slim? Maybe not! Her smile faded away when she saw the price below, '2500 rupees!' She did not have that kind of money. Her Pocket money would total up-to only 500 Rupees. She started sobbing. She will never become thin. All girls were thin except her. She was the only one who kept piling on weight. Tears were streaming down her face. She quickly shut off her laptop.

Chapter 11

Brain explosion

****

An automatic door opened and the vegetables entered the brain from the left side. The leftern hemisphere was known as land of logic and reasons.

The Insides of the brain was bustling with activities. Huge workshops were sprawled across the arena. On ground were lying some transparent tubes with its branches sprawling in different directions just like how roots of trees would spread out. The tubes were all attached to an information counter. That information counter was swarmed with phone calls.

A spider looking creature was firing away the phone calls on the information counter. He handled it like a pro. Few loaf of white breads paced behind him.

"Spider speaking. How may I direct your call?" The spider creature asked like a business man.

"Yellow. Hi. This is spine speaking. Howdy you? My back is really hurting. I need a balm to calm it down. Can you please pass it?" The spine spoke dramatically.

"I will have your stuff immediately passed through the train."

The spider then threw a golden spark towards the tube lying on the ground. The tube caught the golden spark and that spark flowed through it, towards the workshops. The spectacled spiders working in workshops then processed the spark further.

The phone beeped again. "Hello, Spider speaking. How may I direct you call?"

A crying, screaming voice oozed from it. "I have to complain to you about this stones. They are so evil and they are everywhere. They are hitting and punching everybody. They are blocking every nutrient's way. They are not letting anybody do their jobs. And this horrible little carbon dioxide tried to manhandle me today. I am a lady and I feel assaulted. I am going to quit. I am going to quit" she shrilled. "I am so tired. Do something or else I am quitting my job right today." the lady on phone warned.

"Calm down barrier. I will ask the nose to increase its breathing which will decrease our carbon dioxide. I am so sorry they assaulted you. They will be immediately thrown outside the body. As far as stones are concerned I will ask the entire housekeeping department to immediately cleanse the area of them."

"That's the problem. All the house keepers are too afraid to go near them. One of them was hit on head by the stone and had to be admitted in the hospital and now n-n-nobody is willing to go near them." The barrier sobbed.

"I will have rewards sanctioned out for whoever is brave. That will prompt many to try."

"Hope so." Barrier, said wiping her nose, which had liquid flowing out of it.

"Take rest Barrier. You will feel much better." The spider placed the phone down.

Then a different phone beeped. Only one organ in the body could use that phone.

"Hello!" Spider spoke.

"Yellow. Boom Boom shakes the room." A bouncy voice jumped from the phone speaker.

"Hello Adrenal. How may I direct your phone?..." The spider asked rolling his eyes.

"Nothing man! I am already sooo… happy. Inspite of the fact that nobody really knows my existence. But whatever I am still happy." Adrenal spoke cheerfully.

"Then why have you called?" Spider asked already knowing what he was going to ask for.

"Oh yes! I do have a suggestion though. This human is really sad. Shall I release some of my adrenaline in the blood stream?" Adrenal suggested really enthused with the idea.

"For the hundredth time no. You cannot suddenly release adrenaline in blood."

"Why not?" Adrenal pouted.

"Because if you without any reason release adrenal in the blood this human's heart will race itself to death."

"But I do have a reason. This human is really sad. Don't you want to see her a bit pumped up?"

Spider sighed.

"You are holding up the line." Spider said tiredly.

"But I called you on our direct, special, unique, one-on-one phone. How can I hold it up when it's only made for me?"

"I meant you are holding me up. I have other line to attend to."

"Really?" Adrenals pouted again.

"Yeah."

"Still king Bread ruling the entire brain and body from the desire point."

"Whole Brain yes. Whole body no."

"So you take orders from bread now?"

"Everybody in the brain does."

"So you will follow everything it asks you to do?"

"Yes."

"Even sending the signals of eating loads of bread every day to the mouth and the stomach."

"It does send that signal and I do follow it."

"Do you like it?"

"No. But it's my duty." He replied irritatingly.

"O devil's trap! This body is in mess."

"Indeed. Now good bye!" Spider said before placing the phone down.

The original line of Phone again ranged.

"A little bit of glucose for energy." the leg muscle uttered.

"Out of stock"

"10 grams of vitamin k for kidney" The kidney uttered.

"Out of stock"

"100 grams of vitamin A for vision in eye." The eye ordered.

"There isn't much stock of vitamin A left."

"Then signal the stomach to eat carrots." The eye pleaded.

"Can't do. Bread won't give permission, Sir."

"Then signal Stomach to eat a carrot sandwich. That will work?" Cells of the eyes insisted.

"Maybe."

The red button on the black walkie-talkie of spider started beeping loudly. The loafs of breads from the entrance were calling him on it. The spider quickly pressed the answer button.

"Incoming Nutrients 50%, White and red cells 49%, Glucose level 25%, Cleared and Documented at the entrance." The white bread from entrance informed from his walkie-talkie.

"Bring in." The spider answered back from his walkie-talkie. An automatic door opened. Brown and white Loaf entered. The vegetables hid behind a spare table in the corner to avoid being noticed by the loafs. Along with loafs, large cubes of white glucose, nutrients and particles who had become friends with vegetables in train came bouncing in. They were taken to workshops behind.

The loud booming noise of dream from outside was going down by seconds. The projector which was showing the dreams of double-decker grilled sandwich was slowly dying down. A Faint light of dawn broke through skin indicating it was day now.

The automatic door opened again and one more spider shaped creature yawned at its entrance. He was carrying a tray of glucose and joined the first one at the information table by occupying the adjacent seat. He rubbed his eyes of sleep and yawned. "Good morning?" He greeted the first one. "Been up all night?"

"Ahhhmm busy night. Didn't catch a sleep." The first one greeted back tired.

"Glucose? Breakfast? Food? The second one asked offering his tray of white cubes. "It's dry. I generally like it mixed with water."

"Me too. But we didn't get our water supply yesterday, in spite of placing our orders with the mouth. Apparently there is some water shortage in our body." The first spider sighed.

"Did other organs get water?" The second spider asked curiously.

"Yup .Pancreas got one glass of water."

"I don't understand, isn't first destination and preference always the brain?" The second spider asked confused.

"True that. But pancreas was dehydrated."

The other spider opened its computer, sitting on the counter. A voice spoke from that computer.

"Recalling previous night's thoughts.

At front:-Hunger suppressant Pill's

"Desire critically high

Acceptance from bread"

"Why would bread accept the idea of the weight loss pills?" The first spider inquired.

"The girl is very desperate. Even bread can't do anything." The second spider replied grimly as he threw a light spark towards the tubes attached to table .The message was carried forward toward the workshops for further analysis.

The voice from computer spoke again,

"Second important desire.

Cravings for double-decker cheese grilled sandwich.

Acceptance from king bread for breakfast."

"Typical desire." First spider muttered.

"Typical of Bread to keep forming all these desires." second spider nodded

"Just make that carrot double-decker cheese grilled sandwich." The first spider suggested.

"Okay." other spider replied as he threw another spark towards the tube attached to the table.

The voice from computer spoke again,

"Third important desire

Romantic feelings for Jay.

Non-acceptance from the king bread". The spider pressed the "orange" delete button.

"That's an end of love story even before it began." First spider muttered amused.

****

The vegetables saw a door ajar at the other end of the room. "I bet that's the way to desire point" Nerdy Spinach Leaf muttered under his breath. "I think so too." The wise Bitter-Gourd added after a thoughtful pause. All the Vegetables got up from their position and decided to jump from one tube to another tube towards the door. Little did they know that whenever they would jump on a tube it would ignite a memory in Tee's head.

"I hope they don't catch our smell." Garden peas whispered nodding towards the bread loafs pacing behind the spiders.

"Or see us. We have to be very careful." Nerdy Spinach Leaf stated warningly, as he took a step forward. "Will we have to walk on that root like tubes? Make sure you don't get tangled in it."

"My grandfather's neighbour's roots were like this. His name was Banyan tree. People used to worship him a lot. In fact he was the one who taught me how to extend my roots to drink water from a nearby river of our fields." Chubby Cauliflower ranted. "I used to hate organic compost. But he taught me to eat it. Told me, organic compost though yucky to taste, was much healthier than the tasty commercial compost. He told that was his secret to long age. Might be true, he is still living after 290 years." He continued.

"My mother's roots were precious too. So long, thick and beautiful. Her roots were a beauty amongst all the females," Bitter-Gourd remembered.

"My roots were beautiful too. But do you think right now it is the right time to talk all about this?" Nerdy Spinach Leaf scolded.

"All the trees in our garden had long and dense roots apart from ours. Maybe that's why our roots were cut off." Garden peas said sadly.

"Even my roots were not that beautiful." Chubby Cauliflower added in.

"That's wonderful." Nerdy Spinach Leaf clapped sarcastically for chubby Cauliflower. "But can we now concentrate on moving forward."

"Sure buddy. We can go all Ninja over those tubes," chubby Cauliflower replied enthusiastically.

"No need to go ninja. Just don't be seen."

"Alright" They all chorused.

"Or heard." Nerdy Spinach Leaf muttered sarcastically.

They all moved forward secretly avoiding the gaze of loafs pacing behind the spider creatures and also trying not to get tangled in the tubes. They stepped on the first tube. Tee jerked up. Suddenly she heard the "train whistle" that she always loved. Whenever she visited her favourite aunt who lived in the hills, she took the Toy train to see her. The whistle of train was the music of her favourite cartoon. Tee Smiled at that memory.

The vegetables stepped forward on to the next tube. Lemon dropped his puss on it. A strange burning sensation tingled passed through Tee's body. Tee bit back her tongue in the pain.

"Tsk tsk, Lemon." Miss Lady Leek scolded.

"Sorry" Lemon uttered guiltily, "I will be more careful now."

Nerdy Spinach Leaf then walked on the next tube, others followed him behind. As soon as they stepped on that tube, a faint and blurred image started transforming into a clear picture in Tee's head. Tee could vividly now see her old and weak 3rd grade teacher knitting on her rock chair. A black cat with green button eyes was resting at her feet. She waved at tee, whenever she passed her house. She would sometimes invite Tee to share a cup of tea in her kitchen, and inquire about school. She had just retired and missed the school a lot. She had a kind smile and long white hair. Tee would sit on a chair, fold her legs and talk long about school. Hours passed by as they laughed and made merry. The black cat would lick and purr at her feet. One day the black cat died. The weak teacher couldn't hide her sadness and looked gloomed for days. Tee promised herself she would make her teacher feel better. Tee dug a hole in the earth with a spade and helped her old teacher bury her cat. She soon started asking for money from her mum.

"Please Mommy. Loan me some money. I promise, I will return it back when I start earning." Tee pleaded her mum. Her mum smiled at her and kissed her on forehead, "You are a good kid." Tee then surprised her teacher with a new black cat with green button eyes. Her old teacher's eyes lit up and overjoyed she hugged Tee tightly. Once again her old and weak teacher was very happy. Tee blinked her eyes. A rush of love hit her whenever she thought about that incident. She felt very happy.

Next tube had lots of other tubes knotted in each other. It was a huge tangle. Getting caught in it would be a huge risk. Bitter-Gourd jumped over it to avoid getting trapped. Miss Lady Leek and Mrs Lady Finger caught each other's hand and jumped over it. Lemon and Garden peas too bounced their way over it. Nerdy Spinach Leaf skipped it too. Chubby Cauliflower too tried to skip over it but failed miserably. He slipped right in the centre of knotted tubes. One of his leaves got caught in the densely tangled knots.

A sharp noise of whistles and applaud started booming in the ears of Tee. A Picture of nervous 8year old standing and shivering on the stage started playing in her head. Her heart was beating fast. Did she have a stage fright? Well, that is something she would never know before because this was the first time she was looking at some fifty people looking straight in her eyes, waiting with an anticipated breath about what she was going to sing on the stage. She had started reciting her nursery rhymes days before the competition. She must have spoken it many times before, in front of mirror, while brushing, to her mother, to her teacher, to her pet dog. She knew she would remember the lyrics even if woken up from sleep. And true to that she could recall every single lyric of rhyme even though fifty eyes were looking at her. That boosted her confidence. She could do it. Her friends were cheering from audience. She felt positive. She opened her mouth and started reciting the rhymes. She sang smoothly until she was interrupted by one of the judges. "Honey, you need to sing a little bit louder. We can't really hear you." She smiled kindly. Tee was confused and looked forward to the sea of confused eyes looking at her. Some were cranking their necks forward to catch a word of what she was saying. Her friends from audience were signalling her to be little louder. "High" they were all mouthing her. Once again Tee sang. She was nearly half-way when the other judge spoke up. "Have you ever fought with your sister?"

"I don't have a sister, sir."

"Brother?"

"No Sir, I am the only child."

"Oh Jeez! That's a bummer then. You could have really used that fighting voice." He laughed. Few in the audience giggled too.

Were they laughing on her? She thought she was doing great. Why were they laughing on her then? Tears sprang in her eyes. She ran from the stage.

Tee cracked up at that memory. 'Jeez! She was a silly and incredibly innocent 8year old.' Though she laughed it off, Tee couldn't understand why she was getting a nostalgia hit all of a sudden.

"Gosh! You are really heavy." Nerdy Spinach Leaf stated the obvious as he and Lemon tried to pull back the Cauliflower on his feet.

"God made me that way." Chubby Cauliflower muttered with a straight face. Nerdy Spinach Leaf gave hard pull and a sharp pain shooted in Cauliflower's body. His leaf stuck in tangles was starting to break off from his body.

"Not so hard, you doofus!" chubby Cauliflower winced in pain.

"Hey, don't get rude with words, when we are only trying to help you." Nerdy Spinach Leaf shot back irate.

"Sorry! But that really hurt."

"Maybe we are doing this wrong. Pulling him isn't going to free his leaf." Nerdy Spinach Leaf hissed "Yeah we have to open up the knots of tube." Lemon agreed.

"Guys fast or you will attract the attention of loafs." Wise Bitter-Gourd, who was looking out and keeping a watch on loafs said. They started opening the knots of tube. "Hmmm, this is difficult." Nerdy Spinach Leaf muttered as he tried to figure out which tube should be untangled from which another tube.

After a few mistakes they could finally open up the tangled knots. After a hard labour of three sixty seconds chubby Cauliflower's flower leaf was finally freed. They exerted all their power and pulled Cauliflower back to his feet.

"Phew. That was tough!" chubby Cauliflower wiped his forehead.

"You did no work there, buddy." Mrs Ladyfinger told him off, as she followed Nerdy Spinach Leaf on next tube, a thick and beautifully long one at that.

A multi coloured spark flowed through the transparent tube beneath their feet. "That's one of the most beautiful thing I had ever seen in my life." Miss Lady Leek exclaimed.

"Wonder of the body," wise Bitter-Gourd said amazed.

"It was just like the shooting stars we used to see in the night sky from our garden," Garden peas spoke in.

A bird swooped in from the air and landed on a tree, just beneath the shade of which Tee was hymning a song. She threw back her head and laughed heartily whenever she pronounced a lyric wrong.

“For love of the God, It’s paradise, not paraglide,” her friends teased her.

“I keep forgetting it,” Tee laughed it off. The water in river was calm. The grass was tender and soothing. The air was moist. It was a perfect day for a picnic.

“Common! I know it’s pretty, but we are on a mission.” Nerdy Spinach Leaf exclaimed with urgency in his tone.

“Oh hush! It’s so gorgeous.” Miss Lady Leek clapped with delight looking down at all the sparks floating below in the second last tube they were standing on.

“Yeah, contain your happiness!” Nerdy Spinach Leaf hissed irated, “We just have to jump on our last tube. After we cross that, we can easily get through the door.”

Miss Lady Leek sighed and along with other vegetables stepped on the last tube.

A rush of painful emotion coursed through tee’s heart. She hugged all her friends once-more and promised once-more to stay in touch. She packed away her last trunk in the pick-a-way truck. Her mom opened the car door for her. Engine ignited and they zoomed out from their parking lot. Tee waved out to her friends standing on the pavement. “Good-byes” were never easy, as they said. But they shouldn’t be this difficult too. She saw her country-side house for the last time from the rear-view mirror, before it went out of sight. Tee pondered over the fact that how many of her new friends in the city were not even half nice as her town-side friends were.

Chapter 12

Overdoze

At night Tee dreamt about how a big bottle came to her rescue but instead of snatching it, she kept staring it from a distance. Slowly the bottle became smaller and she became larger. Her dress was starting to tear off. Soon the bottle disappeared and she was larger than the room. She could no longer move because she was stuck between ceiling and the floor.

She woke up with a start once again. Her nightmares were happening recurringly now. Her heart was beating erratically, and sweat started forming on her forehead. She clutched her racing heart and tried to catch back her breath. Those weight pills were haunting her and there was no way she could catch sleep again.

Her throat felt dry. She threw blankets on the floor and she slowly tiptoed towards the door of the room. It creaked open when she pushed it softly. Even the stairs made faint noise as she climbed them down.

She drowned two glasses of water straight in the kitchen and headed back towards the stairs but not before noticing a wallet and a phone lying on the coffee table. She hesitated for a moment, not sure if she wanted to do what she was just thinking at the second. She had never done it before and she knew it was wrong. But she was desperate and that overshadowed her guilt. She swiftly pocketed the wallet and phone in her pyjamas and headed back towards her room.

In her room, beneath the false star ceiling, she punched in numbers of credit card quickly in her laptop. The transaction was successful. Even the mobile beeped a faint yellow light indicating a confirmation message. She swiped the mobile and deleted the message. Her mom would now never know that her credit card had just been used.

That night for the first time in months she could sleep peacefully without any nightmares of pills.

Now all she had to do was to wait for a week for her pills to be shipped.

And that day did come after a week. The postman would bring the parcel to her place in morning. But she only reached the post office in early morning. Instead of waiting for the parcel to be brought to her place and letting her mum know, she went to the parcel herself.

It was a big box covered with brown paper. She carried it all the way to her home. As she knew right before that her mom would not be at home at this time it was an apt time for her to carry the box inside. She used her spare key to open the doors and drop the box on her bed.

She tore open the box and inside was a shiny new bottle of pill with a tin cap. She clapped her hands in delight. She took one pill from the bottle and swallowed it. She was sure these pills were magical and would make her thin in no time.

She quickly hid them in her school bag where her mother wouldn't be able to find it.

The day went by quickly. As instructed on the back of bottle, Tee only took one pill each day in the morning and as it was claimed she saw incredible results. On the first day itself her hunger was successfully suppressed and she had not eaten anything throughout the day. Even the night went by peacefully.

Few days went by. She was so happy looking at herself in the mirror. She had lost oodles of weight. She was so happy with her results. She was barely hungry now and was hardly eating anything. She did not even crave food even at night.

But she was still not satisfied. She wanted to lose more weight. She was not happy about the fact that her jeans still failed to fit her.

She took out her pills bottle and instead of taking one she took two. More pills meant more weight loss right?

****

The vegetables finally reached the door on the other side. But sadly as soon as they opened it, they came face to face with the mighty king bread himself. After a few moments of staring at each other in shock, King bread was the one to finally break the silence.

"Well, well, well." the King bread clapped astounded. "Look who decided to pay us a visit. The protectors themselves! The mighty protectors! Wandering in supposedly not their area!" King Bread exclaimed astonished.

"To what do I owe the pleasure of getting a visit from you guys on my land? Though I do have a complaint?" King Bread Pouted "Why have I never been welcomed on your land?"

"Well we..we..ee…are..jus…" Lemon strutted, his puss now dripping on floor continuously due to nervousness.

"Come on let's discuss it in my van." King bread cooed as he gestured his guards to escort the vegetable troop to his van. Big loafs of bread stood in front of vegetables and started pushing them towards the van. When they refused and struggled to get in the van, the guards mercilessly dragged them inside the van. The van was ignited and a huge smoke densed in front of their eyes. All the vegetables coughed in disgust. King Bread took his place in front seat and looked ahead on the road. While the driver loaf sat beside him, all his other guards took the back seats. All the vegetables were sandwiched in middle.

The van soon started moving on the roads of the brain. They passed the various workshops which had an image of some weight loss pill bottle hanging in air. It was a glossy image of small bottle with a tin cap.

King Bread who wore a long cape of orange colour and a crown jewelled with rubies on his head, looked at the pill bottle in disappointment. He was scared, vegetables could sense that. All the spiders inside the workshop rooms were in intense discussion regarding the pill. They all looked dead serious as they examined the pill bottle suspended in the air. A huge message along with pill bottle was also displayed in air.

"Reduce appetite, making you feel fuller, so that you eat fewer calories."

One pill every day before the lunch and the dinner for desirable effects.

- Side-effects Of Caffeine: - high amount of caffeine can cause: - Anxiety, insomnia, irritability and other symptoms.
- It is addictive.

Disclaimer Note: Industry sponsored.

Paid and dubious testimonies.

Not under doctors supervision.

Unauthorized and unlicensed dealer

"LOGICALITY:- ILLOGICAL."

THOUGH ILLOGICAL; DESPERATION LEVEL HIGH

VERDICT: - "YES."

All spiders looked sad when they had to press the green button for approval.

"Something's are still beyond my control in this female's brain. I wish I could eradicate those pills from the face of the Earth. They are a threat." King Bread said angrily to his loaf driver, who was wearing a crisp black jacket and red and white polka tie.

The loaf driver nodded his head in agreement, "But sir, Can't you control her urge to have pills from the desire point?"

King bread bobbed his head 'no', "I tried to empty her head of fashion and boys every day and just concentrate on eating bread. But she somehow manages to refill her brain again with that. And then she wants to become thin to impress them. Now it is beyond my control."

All vegetables in the backseat looked at each other and smirked, well something's were still beyond the control of even bread in brain.

They were now fast approaching the desire point. The point where King bread had placed his throne so that he could control the desires of the entire body. But soon they passed the fort of desire point and that left the vegetables in confusion. If not at desire point then where was he taking them?

Nerdy Spinach Leaf sucked his face in as soon as he realised King Bread was taking them to "Memory loss chamber". A chamber where they would be locked forever if not remembered by the girl within a week. He looked at others in panic. Even wise Bitter Gourd and lemon looked alarmed. Seemed like they had sensed the predicament too. Though these vegetables were alarmed, others were still busy in their own world. Chubby Cauliflower and Mrs Lady Finger were looking in each other's eyes. All three Garden Peas were talking to each other in their pod and Miss Lady Leek was busy judging the amount of smoke the car was creating. Soon they reached the memory loss chamber. The faces of vegetables, which were in their own world dropped on the floor when even they realised what was happening. They too were now on the same page as of Nerdy Spinach Leaf, wise Bitter Gourd and lemon.

The van stopped in front of a door. The guards got down from the back of the van and tried to pull open the middle door of van where the vegetables were seated. The vegetables started pulling the same door from the inside. They refused to let the door open, no matter how much the guards pulled from outside. Finally after exerting all the force they had, the guards flunked open the doors. All the vegetables tumbled down from the car as soon as the doors opened. They were then dragged inside the chambers. King Bread looked at all the antics of vegetables with amusement. He soon followed them inside the chamber and stood in front of them.

"Pray tell me why did you all choose brain as your next vacation spot?" The king bread asked them in determined, yet playful voice.

"Because you kidnapped our beetroots again." Chubby Cauliflower spoke angrily as he tried to kick off the guard holding him tightly.

"Liar-Liar" King Bread laughed it off.

"This is not a joke," Chubby Cauliflower grimed, tightening his hands in a fist.

"Shhh…Shush!" King bread drawled, flipping his hands. "Nobody likes to crack this kind of joke. But if she really was with me, wouldn't I be romancing her in my chambers right now?" A look of pure lust overshadowed on his face "instead of wasting my time here with you."

Everybody's face fell down.

"Thought so!" He taunted calmly before turning his back and descending towards the door with his team of Brown and white loafs.

"By the way I have gone back to my ex-girlfriend Butter. We make a great pair. People like us. We have won people's choice award, plenty of times."

"And", He added

"Make yourself comfortable. It's your home now." He cooed before slamming the door shut. They could hear the keys locking the Lock. They were now locked.

"Are we going to be locked here forever?" Garden peas asked worried.

"If the human remembers us within a week, we will be freed; otherwise we will never be recovered from here. We will be lost over here till the day we eventually perish." Wise Bitter Gourd informed the peas.

"Omg! We are doomed!" Miss Lady Leek exclaimed. "We have opened a trouble box; this human will never will never be able to remember us."

"My son!" Mrs Lady Finger sobbed, "He will be alone and helpless."

"Stay strong! We will get out of here," Chubby Cauliflower consoled, gently stroking her cheeks. She laid her head on his shoulders.

"And I think I have figured out a way!" Nerdy Spinach Leaf cried out thrilled, taking in the surrounding. His eyes wandered on all the crystal balls of remembrance lying in heaps on the grounds. "This remembrance might have our memories."

"Of course they will. This remembrance has been dumped over here by king Bread to wipe out all our memories. If we keep playing the correct one, the human will eventually remember us. That's genius!" Bitter Gourd exclaimed ecstatically and patted Nerdy Spinach Leaf on back.

Miss Lady Leek clapped her hands in delight.

"Now we have to play a remembrance which contains the memories of us." Nerdy Spinach Leaf added attentively.

Mrs Lady Finger walked towards the pile of remembrance on her left. She picked up a crystal clear globe placed abandoned at the top of the heap. She cleaned the fungus growing on it by rubbing her hands on it. She twisted the iron key attached at the bottom of the globe. The remembrance glowed a faint pink in the dark as the key began to untwist itself.

A vague picture started floating in Tee's memory. Hair was ruffling in the wind. A man was wearing grey vest inside a black jacket. His toned arms were handling the bike. His muscled legs were on the pedals.

"Ahh!!" Garden peas, Miss Lady Leek and Mrs Lady Finger sighed together.

"He is gorgeous!" Miss Lady Leek said with a set of dreamy eyes.

"And has gorgeous hair!" Garden peas added wobbling and jumping excitedly on top of each other.

"He is Russell Muscle from the movie Buster Muster," Mrs Ladyfinger piqued in "I happen to know this movie. It was playing on the TV the day before we entered the body.

Miss Lady Leek and I even talked naughtily at what a Catch he was!" Mrs Lady Finger added in shyly, her face turning red from blushing profusely. "I was even married then."

"Alright! Move on to the next one!" Chubby Cauliflower spoke irritated.

Meanwhile Tee wondered where she had seen the picture that had just been played in her mind. She sure knew the man.

Mrs Lady Finger picked up another remembrance lying next to the previous one. She again brushed off the fungus growing on it and twisted the iron key on its base again.

An aroma enveloped tee's senses. She immediately recognised the aroma. It was still her favourite. The aroma of Wet Soil! When she was young and when it rained, she loved dipping her nose in potted plants planted in balcony. She loved taking in the fresh, delicious and cool scent of mud soaked in water by rain. It was a moment of pure joy for her.

"FOOD!" All the vegetables screamed delighted as they saw the soil in the plotted plant.

"Aa!! That looks absolutely delicious!"

"My mouth is salivating."

"Reminds me of the time when we used to feed on pure organic soil boosted by the nutrients of natural fertilizers from the nearby latrines." Lemon remembered.

"And those little earthworm and butterfly family playing circles around me in the garden. Though those bees circling on my head were a tad bit irritating. They were always biting us." Garden peas ranted excitedly.

"Lucky you! The nasty earthworms and rats living in a hole beside me would never leave my leaves alone. They would eat my leaves. It was a big pain for me to re-grow them again and again." Chubby Cauliflower grieved.

"I grew up on black soil in my pot. Excellent soil! It is the reason why I am so smart." Nerdy Spinach Leaf said pushing up the glasses proudly from the tip of his nose. "Though excellent soil also meant lots of microbes and earthworms. But I was an expert in invading them."

"Well my soil was full of pesticides. I have nothing to be proud about," Mrs Lady Finger said making up a face.

"I grew up on red soils of Himalayas. Nobody would even come near me," wise Bitter-Gourd said happily. "My smell is bitter." He added proudly.

"Well and the taste too, the humans would hardly dare to bite you." Nerdy Spinach Leaf teased.

"Their loss." Bitter-Gourd grinned back.

"Well that was quite a useless globe too. We need a globe which will bring back our memories for-god-sake. Not of some soil and food!" Miss Lady Leek said sarcastically. A deep hurt ran through her as she had grown up artificially in a laboratory.

She went ahead of Mrs Lady Finger and picked up another rusty abandoned globe from the heaps.

"Fruity jams!" they all screamed disappointed and put the globe down. Suddenly Tee craved for sugary fruity jams.

"Next better be about us!" Mrs Lady Finger said with her fingers crossed.

"It will be." Chubby Cauliflower winked and Mrs Lady Finger blushed profusely.

Next globe dispensed a foggy air in the crystal. Thunders vibrated. The rains were torrential. A cold current passed through tee's body. The vegetables shivered from a cold wind.

A bicycle zoomed full-speed in globe towards them. The 13-year old rider in it was dripping in water. But she seemed to be enjoying the rains. But her vision was blurring and she couldn't see much ahead. She was failing to see the fence ahead or the bunch of Cauliflowers rooted in grounds besides it. She pedalled aggressively in the direction of fence. She blinked vigorously. She could now slowly make out the shape of fence. She immediately applied the brakes. But Alas! It was too late. She tripped over the bunch of Cauliflowers and the tar wire from the fence pierced sharply across her face. A deep gash ran through her cheeks. Blood started oozing from it.

A pierce pain shot across Tee's body. Automatically her hands touched the scar on her cheeks. She smiled. Though it had pained her years back on that particular day, the wild cycling had made up for it. And rains always had the ability to make her go mad with pleasure. It's been years since she had actually enjoyed any real rains. Now-a-days she would just listen to rain sounds on her mobile apps. But what she could not fathom was why all of a sudden she was bombarded with previous memories.

All eyes turned towards Chubby Cauliflower and stared at him sternly.

"Can't your family not be that clumsy, ever, even if it is just for a bit?" Mrs Lady Finger asked sternly with her hands on her hips.

Chubby Cauliflower ruffled his leaves sheepishly. But suddenly something stuck him. "Hey, but the memory contains me."

"Oh Yes! How could that not strike me?" Nerdy Spinach Leaf exclaimed with wide eyes.

"That's a very well thing then." Wise Bitter-Gourd added, "I Guess."

"We will play this globe again and again till we don't get pulled out of this chamber." Nerdy Spinach Leaf clapped his hands excitedly.

"And then we will finally be able to put this nightmare behind us." Lemon added; suddenly feeling exhausted from all the drama. All of them gathered around the globe and twisted the key again. The scene started repeating in tee's head.

The same mental image of Tee 'riding a bicycle in wild rain' kept floating in her head. Though pleasant memory; the same re-occurring memory was giving her pains. It was now getting very unpleasant. She shook her head aggressively, once or twice, to shrug off the memory. But the memory wouldn't stop playing itself in her brain.

Back in the brain after the vegetables played the memory twice, a violent jerk threw the vegetables on the grounds of the chamber. Nerdy Spinach Leaf tried to find his spectacles which flew from his nose. The globe was still intact in his hands. "This isn't working. It's just giving her tremendous pain in head." He said after finding and re-adjusting his spectacles on his nose. He blinked vigorously to re-gain his sight.

"And apparently causing earthquake in here." Miss Lady Leek exclaimed calmly trying to regain her lost posture. Lemon rolled back to his prior position after rolling around here-and-there; also leaking his puss everywhere he went.

"She is shaking her head to remove the pain and that is what causing earthquakes over here." Nerdy Spinach Leaf straightened it out.

"Maybe you are not that strong enough in the scene to pull us out of the room," Wise Bitter-Gourd said disappointed to chubby Cauliflower.

"I hurt her in the scene. And I am not that important!?" Chubby Cauliflower asked unbelievably.

"Yes, the torrential rains and the joy of bike ride have overpowered you hurting her," Wise Bitter-Gourd added.

"That's a bummer." Nerdy Spinach Leaf said dejectedly, as he threw back the globe in the heap and picked another one. He started twisting the keys of that globe too.

A giddy and tingling feeling shot through tee's body. She remembered a cute guy she crushed on. It was his first day at school. Deep-set eyes, a sharp angled face and a triangle smile with a spaced-tooth. He was shy and just blushed nervously as Tee freely flirted with him besides his locker. If Jay wasn't uncomfortable before coming to school on the first day, he sure was now. He looked down shyly at the floor; His dimples flashed as he smiled, trying to avoid tee's eyes.

Their friendship grew. They started sharing lunch-boxes. Cracked horrible jokes and one day Tee just kissed Jay on his lips.

After that the thoughts of Jay was replaced by fashion in Tee's head. She unnecessarily started worrying about her weight. She drifted away from him. He would often ask her to share the table with him in recess but she would now prefer to share the table with thin girls. They would hardly eat anything from their lunch-boxes and she would hardly eat anything from her lunch-box. Eventually she stopped talking to Jay and would just smile at him if they caught each-other's eyes in school corridors.

She looked back diagonally towards the boy on her left. Jay smiled and raised his eyebrows curiously. She smiled back and looked ahead. He was still incredibly cute. Where were those days when she used to dream about boys? She hardly felt any boy-rush now. She sighed.

"Aww! Weren't they cute while they lasted?" Mrs Lady Finger cooed to Chubby Cauliflower. He smiled back lovingly and clasped their hands together. "Indeed my love! Indeed."

Miss Lady Leek picked up the 6th remembrance ball for the day. As the key untwisted itself, a shrill voice of bell rang in the air. A young frightened girl shivered. It was her first day in the new school. She looked at other kids walking towards the class. "What if nobody talks to me?" Young Tee asked her mom with wide eyes and scared voice. "What if they are mean and bully me?" Her mom crouched in front of her and whispered in her ears, "Be kind and nice. Everybody will love you."

And true to those words Tee managed to make two friends on the first day itself. All she did was "be kind and nice." But that relief was short-lived, because very next day, she had a bunch of test. She didn't want to come across as a dumb new girl in her new school. She wanted to ace it like she always did in her previous school. She cried in evening before the test, when she couldn't complete her lessons. Her mother held her hands while she studied throughout the night. That memory brought tears to tee's eyes. She used to be close to her mother. Now she just fought with her. Now-a-days her life was limited by obsessing about weight loss or thinking about fitting in to the dresses or comparing herself to her Girl-friends. She shrugged that sad feeling off and glanced at the pills in her bags. She was more than determined now to lose all the extra-weight.

"Sweet." Ms Miss Lady Leek said with tears in her eyes, "I might be born and brought up in a laboratory. But I understand what human feelings are", she wiped her eyes, "they are full of intense drama."

"I am a terrible mother who chose to be away from her son for so many days" Mrs Lady Finger sobbed.

"You are doing this only to protect him." Chubby Cauliflower said caressingly.

"We need beetroots to keep this body, our home, existent." Ms Miss Lady Leek said encouragingly, putting her hands on her shoulder. "We need to save his home."

"That's true!" Mrs Lady Finger said suddenly, mustering up courage, "I am doing this only for him."

"Well! That's sorted out then!" Nerdy Spinach Leaf spoke casually, "We can now move on to our next remembrance ball."

Others nodded and encircled Nerdy Spinach Leaf, to look inside the next globe. Loud cheers cheered in the globe. Everywhere adrenalin was pumping in air. Horn blew. Race started. Tee lunged forward in her track. She glanced nervously at her fellow runners on track. Everyone had sprinted ahead of her. She grew her speed a little faster. She could see a faint orange candy in distance. It wasn't that far now, was it? She once again glanced sideways. She could see everyone's back ahead of her. Few had already reached the orange candy and were now plucking it with their mouth. She was still the last. Joining them after a few seconds, she started tucking at her own orange candy secured by clips. She pulled it off quickly with her mouth in a single swipe. She now focussed on the red flag in distance and sprinted right towards it. The wind blew her hair. An excited rush spiked in her body as she ran. Soon she passed the red flag. She looked at her side and saw a boy grinning at her. She looked behind. Most were still pulling at their candies, while others were trying to reach the red flag. Had she secured a second place? She looked around dazed at all the parents cheering her. She had, hadn't she?

Tee would vouch positively about how that particular incident worked wonders for self-esteem of a 9-year old. It also taught her to enjoy sports rather than losing joy in being competitive. Sports and exercises had always been pure fun after that.

"Well this human never ate us. How is she going to remember us?" Mrs Lady Finger snarled irated. Nerdy Spinach Leaf threw the globe back in pile dejected. Wise Bitter Gourd picked another globe from the pile, "We have to keep trying" he said, while handling it over to Nerdy Spinach Leaf. Nerdy Spinach Leaf sighed and twisted the key.

The key started untwisting itself. A 4-year old drooled over which colour is green inside her crayon box in the globe. Her teacher had taught her but she yet again forgot. She re-adjusted the butterfly clip in her hair for the ninth time. Finally after brooding for-a-while she picked up a crayon and started colouring the drawing in her sketch book. She kept murmuring "Lady-Finger", while she covered all the white space within the black outlines of the drawing. She next coloured a bunch of leafs tied with a small rope. She murmured "spinach" while she splattered her same crayon in it. She made a pouty face, when some of it went outside the outline. She then picked up a yellow crayon from her crayon-box. "My favourite colour!" she cried delighted. "Lemon" she squealed, as she pressed her favourite crayon hard, inside the patch of round shaped ball drawn on the paper.

"Alas! It's us!" They all exclaimed excitedly as soon as the globe started playing a video. "Praise the lord!" Miss Lady Leek cried.

"That's perfect! That's our free-us-from-this-jail card!" The garden Peas bounced on top of each-other in their pods.

"And for me, I-might-see-my-son-again card" Mrs Lady Finger chirped in delightfully.

"And to flourish our new relationship!" Chubby Cauliflower winked, as Mrs Lady Finger profusely blushed.

"That's super. Now what's our next step?" Lemon blurted.

"She was young and hence might have problem in remembering us. Now we keep playing it until her memory is clear. She will shake her head to remove the memory from her head but we will still keep playing it until we are eventually pulled out from this place." Nerdy Spinach Leaf hollered. Everybody asserted affirmatively.

****

Tee's mind kept bringing up a vague picture of a box of crayons and a sketch book. She had seen the book before but she couldn't exactly place her finger where. She kept shrugging that picture off by shaking her head. She tried to place that picture at back of her mind, but her mind kept bringing up the picture in front. The picture was blur and supremely unclear. She could just faintly make out the outlines of a sketch book and a crayon-box. She took a pill from her pill-box and gulped it down with water. The pills were working like magic. She was hardly hungry and hence didn't need to eat anything. She smiled at her friends, as she walked up to their spot under tree for lunch, near cafeteria. "It's a bright sunny day and I have smoothies for everyone!" J hollered.

"Yay. That's awesome" everyone exclaimed delightfully.

"I won't drink. Smoothies have 250 calories on average." Tee blew off the offer.

"Well, that's true!" J nodded.

"I will pass too. I had have piled on a lot during the winter." M said exasperated.

"But where's your lunch box, Tee?" J asked curiously.

"Crash-Diet" Tee spoke uncomfortably.

"Good for you. You really need it." J said encouragingly, "I would be so proud of you, if you manage to not eat for at-least for 2-weeks." J hugged her. Tee gave her a half-smile.

****

Lemon rolled around knocking up Garden Peas on his way. The Garden peas laughed with delight. "Once More" the Peas yelled to lemon.

“These damn earth-quakes again!” Chubby Cauliflower spoke angrily as he tried to pull himself up after falling down on the brain floor with a force. He then helped Mrs Lady Finger to get up on her feet.

“She is trying to shrug off the memory again.” Nerdy Spinach Leaf said as he searched for his spectacles on ground with the globe in his other hand.

“It’s quite Ironic! You help brighten vision and you yourself have spectacles” Wise Bitter-Gourd joked. Nerdy Spinach Leaf laughed along with him, “pretty ironic!”

Lemon rolled back in direction of Garden Peas, “Knock you out!” He yelled. The Garden peas giggled as they fell down and tried to bounce back again on top of each out after crashing down from the blow.

“Don’t touch me.” Ms Miss Lady Leek screeched as she jumped of lemon’s way, “Your skin is too acidic for my delicate skin.” She said horrified.

Nerdy Spinach Leaf played the memory again.

Tee again remembered the same scene. She again shook her head

Another jerk tremble the chambers and they all once again they fell down violently.

“No matter what happens, keep playing the memory,” wise Bitter-Gourd advised from the corner he fell down in.

****

At night, no matter how many times, Tee shrugged off the image of a crayon box and a sketch book; it would pop right back in her head. She had definitely seen the book before. Probably when she was a toddler! She had never sketched or coloured anything after turning a teen. She could now though see the vegetables in the picture since the blurred image was slowly becoming clearer. She looked down at her weighing scale. A huge grin broke out on her face. She had lost 2 pounds. She had not eaten anything that day and she wasn’t hungry at all. It was amazing what she achieved by just eating those two pills throughout the day. But that didn’t stop her from dreaming about hot molten cheese melting on toasted bread. But occasionally her hot cheese and bread dream would be interrupted by images of a young girl colouring in her sketch book. It was getting frustrating now. That image was not going to go anywhere. There was no point in even shaking it out now.

"Play it again," wise Bitter-Gourd spoke sportingly for the hundredth time.

"Alright" Nerdy Spinach Leaf said tiredly in a small voice. He was very sleepy.

"And look now the room has stopped shaking every time you play." He added cheerfully trying to keep up the positivity of the room. Everyone else had gone to sleep.

"Do you think we are going to be trapped over here till we perish? Nerdy Spinach Leaf asked gloomily.

"Her memory regarding the incident is very weak, but the image popping in her vision is becoming clearer to her after every time you are playing it," wise Bitter-Gourd said hopefully. "So hopefully we won't be trapped over here till we perish."

****

Tee woke up with a grumbling stomach. She looked at her stash of pills. She decided to take 2 pills that morning though it was clearly disclaimed at the back of the bottle 'not to take more than one at a time.' But more pills meant more weight loss, right? She quickly brushed her teeth, bathed and dressed up for the school. She even quickly shoved the breakfast in the garbage bin while her mom was distracted.

"You forgot your tiffin box yesterday." Her mom spoke, while she closed and packed her tiffin box in Tee's school bag.

"Don't worry about it" Tee said, eyeing the tiffin box the whole time, "I ate pizza from the cafeteria." Now she will have to shove the contents of that tiffin box in her school garbage bin. Her friends might witness it, but luckily they were fully supportive.

"You sure nobody wants to eat this?" Tee asked her friends again as she emptied her tiffin contents in school garbage bin while nobody else from the school was there to interrupt her.

"Nope, Thanks. It looks very fattening." M spoke grossed out. They all walked towards their table and took their seat.

"Yeah M would rather have her spinach salad then the greasy stuff you are carrying." J said, mocking tee with a disgusted face.

"You can share it with me." M said sprinkling her spinach salad with lemon drops.

That's when it hit Tee, When she was young she had a sketchbook which contained drawings of Spinach and Lemon. And one more thing, what was it? Oh yes Lady Finger! She remembered that sketch now. Instead of green she had used pink colour. Her teacher had scolded her for not remembering the green colour again. Tee snorted at that memory.

At the end of the lunch she looked at the clock watch hanging on the wall. It was the time when she took her pill again. Again like morning she decided to take two instead of one. "Umm, what's that?" J asked as she saw Tee removing two pills from a box and gulping it down with water. "That's my new magic potion for losing weight." Tee whispered back scandalously. She was completely sure J would support her. J raised her eyebrow, "Did you consult a doctor before taking it?"

"What's there to consult? The instructions are given right behind." Tee answered back carefree.

"That's because some of these pills are scam. You should not take them unsupervised." J said with a serious tone.

"They are not a scam. I have already lost loads of pounds in all these day. They are really working great." Tee shrugged.

"Yeah sounds scary." M interrupted in sceptically.

"I thought you guys would support me." Tee shot back angrily.

"We are all cheering for your weight loss, but if you are taking pills, somebody from your family should know about it." J said seriously.

Anger rose in Tee. Her head started spinning. Black spots started filling her vision. Things became blur and unclear. "Well this is the only way I am losing weight. You guys need to decide whether you support me or n…." But before she could complete her sentence her head started paining and tears started streaming down her cheeks. She stood up from her chair and walked away from her friends. None of them bothered to go behind her.

****

"We are so stuck!" Miss Lady Leek snapped. "We are never getting out."

"We will have to find another memory which won't be so weak in her memory." Nerdy Spinach Leaf said exasperatedly.

"We have to keep trying. We have to check every Remembrance ball," Wise Bitter-Gourd said determined.

Miss Lady Leek looked around the room. There were heaps and heaps of globes in every corner of room.

"We won't be able to complete every globe in remaining days." She panicked.

"We will. We have to. Everyone pick up different globes and check them quickly. And bring the ones which contain us, right in the centre," Wise Bitter-Gourd ordered.

"That will make the human go mad." Lemon argued with Bitter-Gourd.

"Yeah that will make her hallucinate different memories at once." Spinach leaf agreed along with lemon

"We have no choice." Bitter-gourd said helplessly. He was quite aware that playing different balls at once can make the human go crazy.

Suddenly the doors of the chamber flung open and all the vegetables were sucked out of it. They were flying in air, and before they knew they were being thrown down on the grounds in some other part of the brain.

Chapter 13

Eyes...!!!!

The vegetables ran, scared for their life. They didn't want to end up in the little memory loss Chamber again. They managed to escape this time but weren't sure if the human will remember them again by playing the remembrance once more. The human would never be able to think about them again. It was so sad because they would be so helpful to her body if she would just eat few more of them.

The breads were hot on their heels. Vegetables could see they were not that far behind. They turned in a tunnel at their right. A small door was sitting right at the end. It was a discussion room. They pushed it open to enter inside.

Inside the room few spider detectors sat at a table, looking curiously at an object hanging in the air by projectors. The lady spider cranked up her chin forward to have a better look at the object, "Is that a jewellery box? I can't spot any ornaments in it." She queried curiously.

"Mam, I guess that's because it's not open yet." Her assistant spider addressed her query immediately.

"Uff! It's so blur. My eyes are getting watery just staring at it so hard!" Lady spider said as she tried to figure out the object on the projector. "What does our past experience say?"

"They say it could be a jewellery box but based on past experiences it could also be a textbook." The assistant spider spoke quickly.

"Oh yes, yes!" Lady neuron clapped, having her "aha" moment. "Oh Yes! Yes, it could be! After all its school time' isn't it?" She rubbed her finger on her chin to study it further. She called her assistant spider sitting in a chair besides her, "Ask eye lens to focus more on the object. We need to find out which subject textbook, it is?"

"Yes Mam!" The assistant spider obeyed right away, as she got up from her chair.

The assistant was walking right in the direction of vegetables. Lemon quickly went up to assistant.

"Excuse me mam!" Lemon rolled towards her "Can you suggest us a good hiding place? We are trying to run away from some bread thugs?"

"Not now, you nutcase!" she snarled "Everybody orders me around. You think you will do it too." She growled as she kicked the lemon into a nearby hole.

"Hey! Not fair!" All the vegetables screeched as they ran towards the entrance hole of a tunnel which was night dark, apart from a silver wire hanging in the middle.

"Lemon" Miss. Lady Leek screamed in the hole in a non-lady like manner.

'Lemon'

Apart from her own voice echoing back, she could hear nothing.

"There is no response from lemon." She said confused to others.

"We will have climb down to get him back." Nerdy Spinach Leaf orated as he flung himself downwards on the silver wire.

As he climbed himself down from the wire others soon followed his actions.

"That's very unlady like! I don't like the idea of positioning my legs like that." Miss. Lady Leek said in her British accent, gulping down the awkwardness.

"Do you want to wait here?" Mrs. Lady Finger suggested, "While we get him back."

Miss. Lady Leek looked around hesitantly towards the busy spiders, trying to wrap their heads around the next object on the projector, "an image of some man".

"Is that the Satyagraha dude?" Lady spider asked dubiously.

"That's definitely the Satyagraha dude!" The spiders were busy discussing amongst themselves.

But her eyes soon met the eyes of the evil assistant, who was back in her chair and was once again acting like a civilised person.

"No, I would rather come with you." Miss. Lady Leek cried softly as she turned her body downwards and placed her legs uncomfortably on the silver wire to climb down the tunnel

****

Meanwhile below the wire, lemon stumbled upon rays of sunshine. And in that sunshine he thought his yellow skin looked like Golden Flowers.

****

"This is tiring!" Mrs. Lady Finger said tired.

"Yes! It is a bit difficult!" Chubby Cauliflower said placing his one leg below the other to climb down. His face turned into a painful concentration as he exerted all his strength.

"And how about Miss. Lady Leek? How is she coping up?" Wise Bitter Gourd asked curiously. His voice echoed throughout the tunnel. They were now deep inside the hole.

"I am okay." She said in a small and hurried voice. She kept pulling down her skirt which kept climbing up her knees.

"We might as well as just swing downwards!" Mrs. Lady Finger exclaimed frustrated.

"No don't do that. That will hurt the silver wire. You know how vital this wire is for eyes, don't you? They carry the images to the brain for identification." Nerdy Spinach Leaf ranted alarmed. "So be gentle to the wire. Don't put too much pressure on it and do not swing violently on it."

"Yes, I won't swing down on it Mr know-it-all!" Mrs. Lady Finger huffed back bitterly.

"The only reason I know it, because we are in eye-zone, which is mostly the place of posting for all the spinach after digestion." Nerdy Spinach Leaf retorted back angrily, "My ancestors told me that."

After that the vegetables were silent their whole journey downward the tunnel.

The silver wire ended in an egg shaped room. Millions of light particles were thrown at the back from front of the room. Lemon was busy shinning in middle of that light.

"Lemon, get away from there." Nerdy Spinach Leaf rushed forward to push lemon from obstructing the path of rays of light. Even Chubby Cauliflower ran behind Nerdy Spinach Leaf to stop lemon, but a bit slowly. He was still out of breath from all the rope activity.

"This is such a chilled room." Mrs. Lady Finger exclaimed feeling instantly cooled as she entered the egg shaped room.

"True that. The air in this room has moisture. At least my skin will get hydrated after all the horrible wire activities." Miss. Lady Leek said, rolling her eyes, not so impressed.

"This is wonders of wonder. Everything pales in front of this place. I always wanted to visit this place. I have read so much about it." Nerdy Spinach Leaf's eyes busted out, like a kid in candy store.

"If I am not wrong, we are in eyes," Wise Bitter-pondered as he saw the intense light coming inside the room from a Black hole. Black hole meant that the girl had black eyes. The light coming from that black hole was blinding everybody.

"Look at all the light coming in. It's like a diamond," Nerdy Spinach Leaf spoke mesmerised.

"Are you insane? It's such a gaudy place." Miss. Lady Leek rattled off disgusted by all the strong light, "type of clothes which half of the world wears!"

"I am sure eyes were an inspiration for cinema screens." Mrs. Lady-finger said wide eyed.

"Yes, my dear Okra's mother. They were absolutely inspired from eyes." Chubby Cauliflower appraised her comment and observation skills.

"Look at all these lights forming a picture of Mahatma Gandhi at the back." Nerdy Spinach Leaf said pointing towards the wall at the back. Everybody gaped as the yellow, green, pink, peach and red colours, which were being formed at the back.

"This light is creating magic in the eyes." Nerdy Spinach Leaf puffed his hands in the air like a magician, to gesture the magic happening. "There is yellow, blue, green and all sorts of other colours."

"The girl is right now looking at a photo of Mr. Gandhi, and that's why Mr Gandhi's photo is being formed at the back."

"That's truly a wonder!" Wise Bitter-Gourd commended, clapping his hand.

"And when lemon was standing dancing over there…" Chubby Cauliflower started. Everybody started Laughing.

"I wasn't dancing." Lemon said sheepishly. "I was just standing….umm…wondering…umm…about things."

"The Girl could actually see the lemon dancing." Chubby Cauliflower laughed.

"Ha! Ha! I am a laughing stock now." Lemon pouted.

"You always were, behind your back." Miss. Lady Leek teased.

"Hilarious!" Lemon spoke sarcastically.

"Time to go back," wise Bitter-Gourd announced suddenly serious. "We still have a journey to follow."

That's true and everyone turned their back to go back to the place from where they had just come. But suddenly the rays of light disappeared and there was a complete darkness. After a few seconds the lights came back.

They again turned their back to examine what had just happened. They saw a huge patch of skin opening and closing over them.

"It's nothing! She is just blinking her eyes." Nerdy Spinach Leaf informed everyone. But soon they saw a huge finger approaching the eyes. It started rubbing the whole eye vigorously. The entire eye chamber shook.

Soon the walls started swelling and turning red. Liquid started pouring in rapidly from the walls of the chamber. The girl was crying. The entire eye chamber was now fast filling up with water. Soon the water came gushing down from walls towards the vegetables. All the vegetables got drenched. The water was flowing from eyes towards the cheeks. All the vegetables too were pushed towards the outside of the eye at a rapid speed. The vegetables soon realized what that meant. That meant they would be soon flown out of the eye and thus body. But their realization was too late.

"Ahhh!!" they all screamed as they flew out of the eye.

"Quickly hold on to the eyelashes!" Nerdy Spinach Leaf hollered at the other vegetables. Water rushed in his mouth as soon as he opened his mouth for speaking.

The black eyelash was rapidly going up and down as the eye blinked. The other vegetables quickly followed his instruction and waited for the black hair to come near them. Soon the black eyelash was close enough for them to jump on it. The vegetables held on to it tightly as it went up and down. They could see the water dripping out of the eyes continuously. Again the same finger approached the eyes and started rubbing it continuously. All the vegetables held on to eyelashes tightly to avoid falling down from the finger attack.

Soon the finger moved towards the eyelashes. Now along with eyes even her eyelashes were being crushed by the finger. Even they started shaking violently.

"Ouch!" Miss Lady Finger winced in pain and her juices started flowing out. Along with her, a bit of lettuce leave of chubby Cauliflower got torn too.

Even though spinach had no juice in body, his leaves got torn.

And it was needless to say that lemon had leaked a lot of his puss; which burned the eyes of the girl a lot. It got redder. All the vegetables could even hear the girl wincing in pain. They could only imagine how badly lemon's puss must have stung her eyes. They all stared at Lemon. He looked down embarrassed.

Soon the finger again came in their sight but this time it came along with a black handkerchief. All the vegetables climbed on the top, towards the eyebrow. But sadly while climbing, Mrs. Lady Finger and Lemon were crushed again. Their juices were all over on the black handkerchief.

"Oww!" Mrs Lady Finger cried in pain and let go of climbing. She fell down the cheeks. After cheeks, she would start falling further down the body and then she would eventually crash on the earth. But thankfully Chubby Cauliflower climbed down from the eyebrow and saved his lady in time before she could crash down on the earth. She was badly injured.

The lemon was not that injured compared to lady finger and he quickly climbed towards the eyebrow. Soon chubby Cauliflower with his Lady in his arms followed him to eyebrow too. All the vegetables rested in the Hairy eyebrow full of dead skin cell for some time. They could sense the girl was getting irritated by their constant movement in eyebrow. They tried to move a little less in eyebrow to reduce the irritation to the girl.

But their relief was soon shortened as the girl then attacked her eyebrow with her handkerchief. All the vegetables gasped and quickly ran back towards the eyelashes. Water was still flooding out of the eyes. She sniffed her nose too. Miss Lady Leek had held on to her eyelash so tightly that the hair broke from its place.

Miss Lady Leek screamed as she fell down in the water flooding from the eyes. Lemon quickly offered his hand to Lady for her to hold on to. But she was a bit reluctant to hold his hand which made other vegetables roll their eyes.

"Don't think much and accept his hands." Mrs. Lady Finger urged the other lady. The Other Lady was getting drenched in water as the minutes passed by. Even the weight of water was pulling her down the face. She finally laid her hesitation aside and accepted the hands of Lemon.

The Lemon tried to pull her up but the force of water was quite aggressive. Other vegetables helped him pull her up too. But sadly her hand loosened and she tumbled down the cheeks.

All the vegetables gasped and quickly climbed down to save her. Leek Lady herself held on to the skin of the cheeks tightly leaving a red mark wherever she held it. She slowly started climbing up with the grip of the skin. Water was running all over her.

Lemon extended his hands to her which she gratefully took it this time. Taking advantages of reduced speed of water, Lemon quickly pushed her in the eyes. Miss Lady Leek fell on the grounds of eye chamber. Soon all the other vegetables jumped in the hole and followed her inside the eye chamber. The flooding in the eye room had stopped. But soon they saw the walls leaking a fresh new set of water. The eyes were tearing up again and they had to quickly move from there.

As every-body prepared to walk towards the path they came from, Lemon remembered his previous discovery.

"I wasn't a total useless coming here first. There is a room, right besides this room. Outside that room is a station." Lemon said proudly

"Ohh yes! It must be the digestive route." Mrs. Lady Finger said, suddenly striking with knowledge.

"You are a genius my darling!" Chubby Cauliflower said, stroking her arms with his fingers.

"Okay. Shut up now." Miss. Lady Leek hissed.

"Whoa! Whoa!" Mrs. Lady Finger exclaimed surprised, "What happened to your perfect British manners?"

"Perfect?" Chubby Cauliflower injected mockingly, "More like annoying!"

"Blew away, the moment I hanged up-side down on that awful silver wire." Miss Lady Leek spoke disgusted.

"I like your new attitude." Lemon said appraisingly to Miss Lady leek.

"Oh please stop! There is already one love story to make everyone vomit." Miss. Lady Leek said scornfully, shooting his hopes down instantly while everyone else giggled.

They entered the next room where drum and drums of water were stored. Walls were wet with water pouring out those drums. The floor was also drenched in water. The vegetables picked up their clothes a little higher to avoid getting them wet. They moved their feet through the ankle-length water.

"Do you happen to know anything about this area?" Nerdy Spinach asked Miss Lady Leek sincerely.

"Why, yes! The skin in this area ages really quickly. This area needs the most Botox." Miss. Lady Leek exclaimed horrified.

"Hmm." Nerdy Spinach Leaf thought as he tried to take in this new piece of information. They soon crossed that room and entered the station.

But sadly many bread loafs were patrolling the station. In fact some of them even saw the vegetables entering the station. The vegetables sensing the danger quickly ran towards another open room in the distance.

****

Has she gone so crazy, that she can actually see a lemon flexing his muscles? Right now her teacher was explaining her class about Mahatma Gandhi. But she couldn't see the book on her desk, she could just see a lemon flexing his muscles. She couldn't even see the pills she held in her other hand. Even her pills looked like a muscle flexing lemon. Even her teacher's face morphed into a muscle flexing lemon until she saw a bunch of other vegetables like Cauliflower and spinach pushing lemon away from her eyes. Was this the side-effects of taking pills? Or not eating? J did say that pills would cause hallucinations. Even her mum had said once that not eating will cause her to see lemons.

Tee could feel intense irritation in her eyes. Something had entered her eyes. She blinked few times. She rubbed her eyes vigorously. She felt her eyes swell. They were becoming red. Drops of tears started escaping her eyes. And before she knew she was full-fledged crying.

She picked up her black hanky from the desk and wiped her eyes. She sniffled. Maybe her eyes had an infection. She again rubbed it vigorously with her handkerchief. Tears were unstoppable now.

She could feel something moving in her eyebrow. Little feet were pattering in her hairy brow. She hit her eyebrow with her black handkerchief with full force. When she pulled her black handkerchief down, she saw some liquid on her handkerchief.

There was also a sharp pull at her eyelashes. Fresh batch of tears started springing from her eyes. After crying a bucket finally her irritation went away.

Chapter 14

Ears.

They all ran as fast as they could with bread loafs hot behind them. They ran from one room to another. They finally entered a room and while running tripped over in a tub filled with sticky liquid. There were small rapid waves in that liquid. The sides of tub were lined by number of small hair. Whenever the liquid moved, it would shake the hair too. The waves in liquid were constantly making the hair on sides move too. And whenever the hair moved, some little flickers of sparks floated in air.

"This liquid is so cool. It's giving me the shivers." Miss Lady Leek grumbled as her teeth started chattering.

"You are so delicate." Lemon cooed.

"Shut it." She snapped "Or I will drown you in this liquid." She said with a thin smile.

"That would be a shame." Lemon muttered clearly embarrassed.

"And why is this liquid creating so many violent ripples? And these hairs rubbing against my arms are going to give me rashes." Miss Lady Leek said annoyed.

"I guess we are in ears." Nerdy Spinach Leaf concluded looking around at the surrounding.

"And the ear has a tub?" Miss Lady Leek asked sarcastically, "Sounds hilarious."

"Oww.....this tub is wonderful!" Mrs. Lady Finger cooed as she enjoyed their sudden bath. "I thought you always liked taking a bath." She added in ears of Miss Lady Leek.

"Not this suddenly. I like to be prepared beforehand. I always add few drops of oil and some salt before taking a bath. Without all that it's just water. And this isn't even water. It's all so sticky..." Miss Lady Leek moaned, hating all the liquid sticking to her like glue.

The sound of sparks buzzing from the tub was loud and clear. Few more sparks sparked in the air from the tub.

"Where are these sparks going?" Mrs. Lady Finger asked in wonderment.

"To the brain." Nerdy Spinach Leaf perceived, "To send the message of hearing. This is real travelling." He added happily.

"Beaches in stomach are travelling. Those famous flower shows in the legs are travelling. That Vast farm in Thigh is travelling. Or that big blood fall in heart is good as travelling. But getting stuck in sticky liquid is not travelling." Miss Lady Leek straightened it out.

"Each to its own." Nerdy Spinach Leaf sighed.

"Well I can't take this hair anymore." Miss Lady Leek said irritated as she got out from the tub. Mrs. Lady Finger followed her. They both wiped out the stickiness on their body. Chubby Cauliflower came rushing from the tub to help Mrs. Lady Finger.

"This hair is truly very irritating." Lemon spoke displeased too and got out of the tub.

"Just like your puss." Miss Lady Leek added in smartly.

"I don't like you anymore." Lemon complained hurt.

"Ooo... should I cry?" Miss Lady Leek cooed.

Even Garden Peas bounced out of the tub followed by the Wise Biter-guard.

Nerdy Spinach Leaf refused to get out of the tub. He was enjoying himself too much to come out but finally when everyone started moving ahead without him, he reluctantly came out. Thankfully for them there was no sight of bread loafs till now.

Ahead was a dark bonny tunnel.

"I wonder where this bony tunnel takes us," Bitter-Gourd exclaimed as all the vegetables moved ahead in the bonny tunnel.

Ahead at the end of the tunnel they could witness a round boxing bag hanging from ceiling. It was light pink in colour and matched the colour of the walls of tunnel.

"Hey it looks a bit like me?" Lemon exclaimed excitedly as he looked over his body, "Just that I am yellow, this is pink." He said adding the obvious things that even others could witness as well. "Also I am not hanged. I wonder why that is hanged." He asked curiously as he walked towards it and punched it.

****

Tee jerked up with a sharp pain in her ears. A buzzing sound was ringing in her ears. She was feeling drowsy before because of exhaustion from all the hallucination in her eyes; but now she was wide awake because of all the piercing pain in her ears. For a split second she felt she wouldn't be able to hear anything. The same sharp pain thundered in her ears again. She gasped in pain. She couldn't hear what her science lab partner was telling her. It was like somebody was mercilessly punching and pulling her eardrums from inside. She pressed her ears on her shoulder to numb the pain.

****

"What are you doing?" Nerdy Spinach Leaf asked as he saw lemon punching and pulling the eardrum.

"I just want to take it down so that we can examine it. I think it's a lemon too." Lemon said obviously.

"No it's not a lemon. It's an eardrum." Nerdy Spinach Leaf fumed back. But Lemon ignored him and punched her drums some more, and then again and again.

"Stop punching her drums." Nerdy Spinach Leaf said irritated. Now he was filled with anger.

"But I am a Lemon and I think this is a lemon too." Lemon shouted on top of his voice.

"Stop shouting because whatever we speak from here, she would be able to hear us." Nerdy Spinach Leaf said frustrated.

"Oh yeah! Then I have a lot to tell her. Why wouldn't you eat us? We are moving earths and mountain over here to save you." Mrs. Lady Finger screamed in Tee's ear drum.

"Sensitively, my dear, eardrums are very delicate." Chubby Cauliflower told her calmly.

"Just push us down your throat." Mrs. Lady Finger spoke again, but this time much more calmly.

"Yes, just eat us." Miss Lady Leek spoke joining Mrs. Lady Finger.

"Eat us! Eat us! Eat us" They both cried and begged now.

"That would be enough girls! I am sure she got the message," wise Bitter-Gourd said understandingly as he knew the sudden voices from inside the ears would panic the child.

****

The pain made her whole ear go red. She pressed her ears with her fingers tightly to numb the pain.

"I am a Lemon. This is a lemon too."

"Stop it! This is not a lemon."

She could hear various voices. She looked around. Everybody was either yawing or had their heads in their book. But she could still hear voices. Who were they? And why would they call themselves lemon. Was she hallucinating again? Was the voice coming from her head? This was heights. Now she was hallucinating a lemon talking. Were these all a side effects of taking pills? Or not eating? Was J correct? Were these pills that harmful?

"Eat us. Eat us. Eat us."

"Push us down your throat."

Eat who? Lemon? Was the food she threw in garbage in recess talking to her? If yes, then from where? Was she going crazy? Has not eating food made her go mad?

She could now hear chairs and tables telling her to eat them. She looked at her surroundings. Even humans were telling her to push them down her throat. These pills might turn her into cannibalism. She should have consulted a doctor before taking them.

Sweat started beading on her forehead. Tee was on the verge of crying. She blinked back her tears. Her head was also paining mercilessly. And periodically her vision would become weak and black spots would start dancing in front of her eyes. First her friends scolded her and now she was hallucinating a lemon walking and talking in front of her eyes and ears. It was abnormal.

"Eww, so much goo! Does this girl even clean her ears?"

Tee looked besides her. Her neighbour girl looked up from her book and smiled at her. She smiled back at her hesitantly. She then turned her head towards her book. But she again heard her neighbour girl speak something.

"Unhygienic girl!"

She looked back at that girl again. Why was she so mean and then pretended to smile at her? Tee checked her arms for body odour. Her arms were fine. She checked her mouth. She had brushed properly that morning. Surely there was nothing unhygienic about her mouth. Tee made a face at that girl. Immediately her neighbour girl stopped smiling at Tee.

****

The tunnel of eardrum turned into a slope ahead. Some yellow sticky goo lay randomly on floor and walls. Some were splattered on the ceiling of the ears.

"I am tired. I am going to climb and lay on the slope for a while." Miss Lady Leek sighed and walked towards the slope, but she slipped on that sticky yellow goo. She fell down right there on her butt. She tried to pull herself up again but her leg was stuck on the floor to the goo. She had a hard time detaching her leg completely from the sticky goo. When she did manage, its bits and particles were still sticking to her feet.

"What is this goo on the slope?" She exclaimed grossed out.

"Goo? That's not goo. That's ear wax." Nerdy Spinach Leaf spoke unbelievably.

"Nasty ear wax seems more like it. It's so sticky." Miss Lady Leek said trying to get rid of bits and pieces stuck to her feet. "Why don't they clean this place? It's so unhygienic!"

"Hardly nasty, it's produced by ears itself to protect the skin of the ears. It traps dust and keeps the ear clean." Nerdy Spinach Leaf clarified.

"Keeping ear clean by spreading its goo on the floor?" Miss. Lady Leek asked unbelievably, "That's ironic!"

"And besides there are commercials of ear buds which clean this goo. I think the girl is just lazy. This is the most unhygienic place on the earth." She continued disgusted.

"Well I think she can hear you." Nerdy Spinach Leaf asked her to lower her voice.

"Well that's good. She should know she has to clean this place." Miss. Lady Leek shrugged casually as she sat down on a clean spot that she could find on the slope.

Nerdy Spinach Leaf sighed and walked forward and climbed on top of the slope, while others just followed him. But sadly they all were slipping on the ear wax and kept sliding off the slope. They had to climb up the slope again. Goo was stuck on their knees and arms. Their finger had gotten sticky. Wise Bitter-Gourd somehow managed to join Nerdy Spinach Leaf on top. Lemon got stuck in the goo while others still kept falling off the slope. The pod of garden Peas had very thin legs and hence could not manage to make his balance on the goo. Same went for Mrs Lady Finger. She too had extremely thin legs. While chubby Cauliflower kept rolling off the goo.

"Why don't you all rest with me?" Miss Lady Leek suggested from where she sat on the slope. But all the remaining vegetables ignored her suggestion and kept trying to climb the slope. Finally they held each other's hands tightly, walked up to lemon and tried to pull him from the goo. They exerted all their force and were finally able to free the lemon from the stretchy and sticky yellow goo.

Once again they caught each other's hand and climbed the remaining slope and joined Wise Bitter-Gourd and Nerdy Spinach Leaf at top.

From top of the hill they could see a faint light coming in from a hole at the end. They could hear a faint noise buzzing from that hole continuously. They started walking towards the hole. The buzzing noise grew louder as they approached the hole. They soon realised it was coming from the outside world. Everybody stood at entrance of the hole and looked around. Chill of air conditioner greeted them. The insides of the body were burning hot and they all felt cool after a long time. The buzzing noise also became more audible. They could see the entire outside world from that hole. They were in a classroom. There were girls and boys with their heads buried in a book, while a teacher was chalking up the board with her handwriting.

"Mahatma Gandhi was the father of the nation." the teacher spoke. Lemon climbed out of the hole and sat on a pointy structure outside the hole. He looked around and saw a group of girls and boys staring at him with their mouths open and eyes wide open. He waved at them. Chubby Cauliflower quickly came out and pulled the lemon back inside the hole. Everyone gasped, as they not only witnessed a Lemon but also a Cauliflower coming out of the ears.

****

Tee was feeling extremely irritated. Her ears were still red and she felt as if something was moving inside her ears. Had an ant entered her ear? It was causing her inside ears to tingle. She shook her entire ear with her finger. For a second the movement stopped but then it started again. She kept jabbing and poking her finger in the ear. And now the movement was quite continuous.

Swiftly a finger came towards the hole and shook the whole ear. Lemon and Nerdy Spinach Leaf fell abruptly outside the hole while trying to get back inside the hole. They were going to get crushed but were saved marginally. All vegetables gestured them from inside, to come in quickly, while they also tried to save themselves from the finger and its sudden shaking the ear. That finger could crush and churn them or probably make a paste of them like a grinding mixer.

Seeing the chance to escape the finger, lemon and Nerdy Spinach Leaf darted towards inside the ear. All the vegetables started running aimlessly and recklessly on the path from which they had come from. Miss. Lady Leek who was busy contemplating between whether she should join others or she should keep seated at her current position saw her fellow vegetables running in her direction. She inquired about why they were running like men on fire, but was only met with a hurried "Run. Attack. Run." reply. She did feel trembles minutes ago, but just passed it off as maybe the human burped.

"Did the human burp? The ears were trembling a few seconds ago." She asked puzzled.

"No, it's a finger attack." Nerdy Spinach Leaf said, not stopping to answer and still running hurriedly towards the water tub. Others followed him, but sadly slipped over the ear wax on the slope. They tried to get up, but another tremble pushed them down the slopes. They tumbled down and fell on their face at the bottom of the slope.

"Finger attacks in ears? Why would a finger again attack in ears?" Miss Lady Leek asked confused as she joined others, as they again stood up after falling down. They somehow managed to pass the Water tub and the followed the electric sparks sparking from the tub. Those sparks would take them to brains.

They all ran towards the brain hurriedly. They then followed the silver electric sparks in to a narrow tunnel which led them back to the discussion room of neurons discussing objects on the projector.

****

Bell rang and class was dismissed. Tee got up from her place and walked towards the hallway. But she could feel few people staring at her weirdly. They looked at her from top to the bottom. Did all of them find her unhygienic? Last checked she had brushed her teeth, took a bath and combed her hair. Then why would they find her unhygienic? She had even washed her clothes before wearing them. Maybe she didn't iron her dress properly. Could that be the reason? A few ripples on her cloth. She couldn't take the eyes gawking at her anymore. It was getting too awkward for her. She quickly moved towards another classroom.

"Maybe it was an earring." The boy whispered.

"It waved to us!" The girl whispered back.

"Maybe we are hallucinating." Another boy added in.

"We all are?" The girl asked shocked.

"She's a freak." The first boy declared.

"Yes she is. I smiled at her and she made a face at me. How mean!" The girl gave her opinion too.

"She was always a freak." Another girl chimed in.

"Look at her ears. They are so red." Another boy observed and stated.

"Maybe she does Voodoo and all." Another girl suggested.

"That's so scary." The first girl said frightened.

"Next we might get to see carrots and potatoes coming out her ears." They all laughed.

Chapter 15

Nose...

In the chamber all the spiders were again in some deep discussion about smells of flower that was currently lingering in air throughout the room.

"I think it is Lilies." The assistant spider said sincerely like how a good assistant spider would say. Only vegetables knew how evil she was.

"No this smell is definitely Jasmine." The lady spider concluded as she took another whiff of scent in air.

"Alright. If you say it's Jasmine, then it's definitely Jasmine." The assistant spider gave the fakest sweet smile before she caught the sight of vegetables in the room. Her fake smile disappeared and she stared at them with all the anger she could muster.

Even the Lady spider sensed the presence of vegetables in the room. She looked at them curiously.

"Where did you people disappear? I have arranged a ride for you guys till station." She informed them.

The vegetables looked at her with wide and happy eyes. They couldn't believe what they had just heard. They would finally be going home.

"That's very sweet of you." Wise Bitter-Gourd came forward to thank her gesture.

"Take a seat till it arrives." Lady spider suggested them to take the seats placed in the corner of the discussion room.

One by one all the vegetables took their seat in the corner. They were grateful that finally they would be able to reach their home back. They had enough of adventure. Coming to the brain, was a waste since they couldn't find beetroot and they were being constantly attacked.

Suddenly Spinach started smiling and jumping happily. All the other vegetables looked at him weirdly.

"Do you know what we are sitting next to?" He asked them excited.

All the vegetables turned their heads to express their 'no'. Some looked at him curiously while others like Lady Leek were purely disinterested.

"We are sitting next to the nose tunnel." He told them delightfully like a jumpy kid.

The ears of lady Leek perked up and suddenly she looked very interested.

"The nose, which has treasure buried in it?" She asked him hopefully. Her heart beats increasing its pace.

"Yes." Spinach replied quickly.

The Lady Leek looked at him shocked for a second but then started clapping delightfully.

"Let's go and find the treasure then." She told spinach with pleading eyes.

Spinach nodded excitedly and got up from his seat. Wise Bitter-Gourd pulled him back quickly on the seat.

"Nobody is going anywhere now." He told to both the Spinach and Leek. "We had enough of adventure."

"I know I want to go home to my son." Lady Finger said tired.

"But we have come so far. Don't you make our trip worthwhile by finding that treasure?" Spinach persuaded and begged them desperately.

"I know our whole trip has been so disappointing till now." Leek added in to persuade them further. "And your son will love those treasures." She told Lady Finger hopefully.

Lady Finger did agree with that part. Her son would love to have been gifted with treasure. Especially after she had told him repeatedly at the bed time, story of how humans dig and poke their nose for treasure.

She looked at Bitter Gourd. The Bitter Gourd looked back at her.

"Alright," he told them and all the vegetables got up from their seats and walked secretly towards the nose tunnel. It was seemed long and thin. Maybe the girl had a pointed nose. Scents of Jasmine wafted throughout the tunnel. Most of them turned their nose upwards to take in the aroma.

"Jasmine flower was once upon a time my girlfriend. Her pot was just besides my pot at my master's place." Nerdy Spinach Leaf spoke nostalgic.

"I feel sometimes he is just making things up." Mrs Lady Finger whispered to Miss Lady Leek.

"Or probably lying, since he knows we don't know anything." Miss Lady Leek whispered back.

"That's what I said" Mrs. Lady Finger whispered again as she turned her nose upwards to take in the smell of rose now.

"Oh! I didn't realize!" Miss Lady Leek bit back her tongue.

As they kept walking deep inside the nose they could see big storms at a distance.

"I must say this place is very well ventilated. There is loads of warm and fresh air." Nerdy Spinach Leaf appraised as they now took a ninety degree sharp turn, and stood on the top of a steep, sharp and pointed slope.

The air which was calm and breezy till now in the tunnel was fierce on the top of the slope. Air was furiously being sucked in and out through the holes of the nose. The air wasn't just warm now but flaring hot. The walls were intense maroonish red on both sides of the slope.

"This is real the nose. This is where the treasure is." Wise Bitter-Gourd informed others. "But to get the treasure we will have to brave this wind" He quickly added.

"I am game. I want that treasure." Nerdy Spinach Leaf said enthusiastically.

"This place is full of treasure. I want them all." Lady Leek said determined.

"I have heard humans aggressively dig this part. I hope there is some treasure left for us in this human nose." Lady Finger added in hopefully.

The wind blowing ferociously was hitting them sharp in their faces.

Chapter 16

The Unknown Treasure

The slope was long and sharp. They were trying to climb down the slope in the opposite direction of the wind. There was also a rush of air, pushing them from behind. First the air from front would slap them right on their face. And then the air from behind would push them forward. They were trying not to lose their footing or skip their feet which would make them fall down the slope and right outside the body through holes of the nose.

"We will find a spot and start digging there for treasure?" Nerdy Spinach Leaf spoke in sore voice as all the wind was making his throat dry.

"What will we dig it with?" Miss Lady Leek asked equally pained by wind hurting her cheeks as she tried to move forward on the slope carefully, braving the winds.

"With our nails," Nerdy Spinach Leaf answered back in his sore voice as he too tried to climb down the slope, "I just hope we are able to notice a perfect spot through this wind."

"Not me. I love my nails." Miss Lady Leek replied cheekily.

Mrs. Lady Finger was the slowest and was left a little behind as the wind was hitting her back and forth. She held the sides of the wall to balance herself; while on the other hand Chubby Cauliflower ahead of her, too, was holding the dark red wall of nose tightly, leaving a minute red swell wherever he touched. To be precise, he wasn't even moving. He was letting the wind from the back push him forward. He thought he was the smartest in their entire vegetable troop for moving ahead like that.

Little hair became more visible on the side of the walls now. They also became more visible on the ground of the nose. Those few hair particles became a lot as they kept going down the slope. But now along with hair there was something else hiding in hair too. Something extremely sticky. It was sticking to their body and it also smelled horrible. They disliked it immediately.

"Eww! What is this goo sticking on my hand? It's so wet and stinking." Miss Lady Leek spoke disgusted to see something sticky stretching on her hand.

"It's booger!" Chubby Cauliflower busted out crying.

"What? That is so disgusting. Just like in the ears!" Mrs Lady Finger said horrified.

"Worst than ears! I take back what I said earlier about ears! This is the most disgusting place on the earth." Miss Lady Leek declared.

"These boogers are everywhere. And they are so big." Lemon spoke astonished.

****

Tee felt something moving in her nose. It was pinching the walls of her nose from inside. The movement in the nose increased. Even the pinching increased. It was now irritating and itching her. She inserted a finger in her nose and started pulling out whatever was moving in her nose. She pulled out her finger and it was just a booger.

****

The light coming in from the hole reduced as a finger approached its entrance. Soon the finger entered the nose and started scraping its ground and the wall. All the vegetables jumped on the side of the wall to avoid the finger. All the boogers started shaking and some even slowly started detaching themselves. The boogers were pulled forward by the finger. The finger finally managed to pull a booger out of the nose.

"This is what the human are always digging!" Miss Lady Leek spoke disgusted; "Boogers!" She tried to get rid of the sticky booger on the wall besides her. It was ready to pop out from the wall anytime soon and fall on her. "I don't want to continue this search anymore." She cried.

"To be precise boogers are nose necessities." Nerdy Spinach Leaf spoke. His legs were trapped in liquid booger. Even one were somehow trapped and touched by boogers, because wherever they went in nose tunnel there were boogers.

"Are you crazy?" Mrs Lady Finger asked irritated.

"Enlighten me," Wise Bitter-Gourd asked curiously.

"No please!" Lady Finger cried. "Nobody wants to know how a booger is a nose necessity." But before she could even finish, spinach had already started speaking.

"To be precise it catches dust from the air inhaled. They are like frogs which catches the mosquitoes. They are like flowers wh..."

"Okay! That's enough information for the day." Mrs Lady Finger stopped him in middle.

Once again the finger entered the nose and right now aimed straight towards the Miss Lady Leek. Miss Lady Leek got scared and pinched the sides of nose tunnel more tightly. The finger touched the tail of Miss Lady Leek and pulled it. Lemon, who was standing just on the top of the Miss Lady Leek, kicked the finger hard. He jumped on the fingers. He kept jumping on it till the finger loosed its grip on Miss Lady Leek. Soon the finger was out of the nose.

"So that's their treasure. They always dig for boogers." Miss Lady Leek concluded once again.

"clearly." Mrs Lady Finger added.

The side of the nose started shaking violently as the girl started poking it from outside. The vegetables had to jump from here and there, whenever and wherever the girl poked. Or else they would get crushed, and it will squeeze out all their juices, and that juice would drip out of the nose.

The whole nose swelled up. It's inside turned intense red. Liquid Water started pumping in the nose from its walls. That water started falling out from the nose. The girl was constantly trying to rub it away.

Once again, she pierced her finger in the nose and this time aimed straight towards the Lemon that was clinging on to a booger on the side of wall.

"Ouch! Get lost! You crazy woman! He kicked and stomped on her finger."

She once again pulled her finger out of the nose but not for long as she once again dipped her finger in the nose and started randomly poking it aggressively everywhere. Every vegetable started running erratically here and there in the nose.

"She's gone crazy." They all shouted.

Suddenly the girl started exhaling very strongly. The wind pushed them strongly from behind. They were all losing their balance.

"If she keeps exhaling like this we all will fall down from the hole," wise Bitter-Gourd said warningly to others.

"This is crazy!" They all said frightened holding on to the walls of nose tightly. Miss Lady Leek held on to the booger, even if she found it disgusting.

Puss of lemon started oozing out. It burned the delicate skin of her nose. They could hear girl hissing and wincing in pain unable to grasp what is happening with her? All the vegetables looked at Lemon sternly.

"I am injured. I can't help it." Lemon looked back at them innocently.

A great flow of water drops rushed down at a lightning speed.

"Achoooo." They all heard and in a minute they were all thrown outside the hole.

****

"Ouch." Somebody is hitting her finger. Also she felt the pinching starting in her nose again.

Water started dropping out of her nose. It was burning and paining her. She quickly pushed her finger inside the nose and started pulling the thing that was pinching her nose from inside. Her whole nose was shaking and had turned red. She kept pulling but eventually only a booger dropped out of her nose. She quickly wiped it with her handkerchief. But it was too late. People had already seen it. They were staring at her in disgust. Some of them even had their mouths open in shock. How could somebody dig their nose in public in this civilised world?

She was truly a freak. An uncivilised freak who digged her nose in public. Bell rang. Class was dismissed. Tee could feel eyes boring on her. They were all gossiping about her. Laughing on her! She could even feel the pinching in her nose start again. It was irritating her now. Tears sprang up in her eyes. She quickly got up and headed towards the washroom.

****

Everybody fell in the direction of hole. But due to high wind all except Lemon were swayed and thrown on a skin plank near the entrance of the nose. Lemon fell right out of the hole. Fortunately Bitter-Gourd standing on the edge of the plank had held him by his hand. The girl's hands caught the Lemon and started pulling it down violently. All the other vegetables helped Bitter Gourd pull the Lemon upwards, back in the nose. Though their strength was marginal in front of her, they were throwing in every strength they had. A tug-of-war broke between them as they both tried to pull Lemon in their direction, while Lemon winced and screamed in pain. Then there was a sudden release by girl's hand and all the vegetable jerked the Lemon back inside the nose. They all panted heavily as they lied on the plank. After couching on plank for a while they decided it was time for them to head back. They decided to quickly climb back the slope since they didn't want to get caught up in another storm which might brew up in the nose. Hence they quickly got up and started moving urgently.

The poking of the finger once again started from the outside. It was like a game as they tried to escape getting squeezed and trying to avoid getting stuck in the booger at the same time. They climbed the steep slope with the help of boogers, the same boogers they disgusted on initially. Many times they would get stuck in a small booger but managed to pull themselves out of it with all their might.

But unfortunately Mrs Lady Finger got stuck in the big liquid booger. At that very moment the girl poked the nose from outside. Mrs Lady Finger was hit by the wall again and again. Cuts and scrapes started forming on her body. Juices started dropping out of her body. Chubby Cauliflower tried to unglue Mrs Lady Finger from the booger whenever he could get the chance. But the girl was continuously poking the nose aggressively. Finally the poking stopped. Chubby Cauliflower carried the injured Lady Finger in his arms and rushed towards the top of the nose.

They finally reached the top of the slope and retreated back on the path from where they had entered the nose. Now they wouldn't dare to explore anything in the body. They all were scared. They would just reach back to the brain, where the spiders would give them a ride to the station. But even before they could take a step towards the brain another sneeze trembled the whole nose. All the vegetables lost their footings and instead of going upwards, they all started falling down in darkness.

****

She exited her class and entered in the lobby. A constant fluid was coming out of her nose. People were staring at her red nose. Then her nose sneezed loudly. More drops of water came out of the nose. But along with water, something yellow also dropped out of the nose. Many people saw that. Their mouths fell on grounds in shock when they realised it was a Lemon. They also saw a Bitter-Gourd pulling the Lemon inside. Their eyes got wide witnessing that.

Tee could see people staring at her with wide eyes. Few were curious. Few were shocked. Others were pure disgusted. Her cheeks were soaked with tears. Her Eyes were still red and her ears were burning red too. She rushed towards the washroom as fast as she could.

On her way she could hear people are laughing on her.

"You have a lemon coming out from your nose." They all informed her.

"You really are a freak!"

She was breathing ferociously now trying to exhale out the thing that was irritating her from her nose. She was looking like a possessed woman breathing extreme heavily. She didn't want to dig her nose in front of everyone again.

In the washroom her reflection of mirror showed a yellow ball coming out of her nose. On a close inspection she realised it was a lemon. She pulled it outside her nose. But something else was pulling it back inside. She could even hear the Lemon screaming in pain. That shocked her. She pulled it outside with much more force but he was pulled back in again. Tee Sighed. This time Tee exerted much more force. She almost succeeded in pulling the lemon outside the nose but then she saw a Bitter-Gourd pulling it back inside. She saw a Bitter-Gourd! She left the lemon in shock and Bitter-Gourd successfully pulled him inside the nose. Tee stood there in bathroom witnessing all this in shock. She had completely gone mad now. She was hallucinating, not just a Lemon but also a Bitter-Gourd now. She immediately searched for pills bottle in her bag. These all were really the side effects of eating pills. She shouldn't have taken them at all and now she was turning into a freak. She flushed those pills into the sink. Finally she felt a little relieved in the whole day. But that was short-lives as she again felt movements happening in her nose again. She again stated poking and pressing her nose. She rubbed her whole nose continuously.

Chapter 17

Ribs.........

Gravity had never made its currents stronger. They were falling down a pipe faster than an apple falling on Newton's head. They were also moving down in heavy air.

"We are flying." Lemon observed.

"Ohh! I am loving it!" Miss Lady Leek clapped her hands delighted.

"This is heaven." Mrs Lady Finger said as they all kept falling downwards in pipe amidst all the gushing winds. At a distance there was a door.

They managed to get hold of the door. That door opened up to a lobby of lung. They all entered the door and fell on the grounds of the lung. They lay still for a moment on the ground. Wind blew above them.

"What do we do now?" Chubby Cauliflower groaned while lying on his back, his voice tired. "This is insane, how do we go back home?"

"We can climb back the pipe or catch a carbon-dioxide train from lung station." Wise Bitter Gourd suggested.

"Monster carbon-dioxide." Garden Peas said snarled.

"No! No! We don't want go on the station. We are again in the same lobby which the Phagocyte patrols. We will never get out of here alive." Nerdy Spinach Leaf cried.

"But if we climb back the pipe we will be back in the sneezing nose. No thank you." Lemon dismissed the other idea too.

"I want home. I miss my son." Mrs Lady Finger spoke sadly.

"I miss home too. Somebody just take me home. I had enough of this nonsense." Miss Lady Leek grumbled.

"Sacrificing myself in digestion doesn't seem like a bad option right now." Nerdy Spinach Leaf Laughed.

The vegetables contemplated their option and catching a carbon-dioxide train filled with carbon dioxide felt like a better option than climbing the pipe and getting sneezed out from the nose.

"Let's head towards the station then." They all made up their mind and headed towards the station.

****

They started walking down the lobby and headed towards the bony stairs which would eventually lead them to the platform.

They saw a Yellow glow from a distance. That yellow glow did not move and stayed in one place.

"Die trespassers! Die" He screamed at them when he saw them. It was phagocyte. All vegetables got scared and rushed in another direction before being stopped by Wise Bitter-Gourd.

"Wait! Wait." Biter-gourd hollered, "Look Carefully. It's tied up." He said.

All the vegetables turned their heads towards the yellow glow and indeed the phagocyte was tied-up. They all stopped running.

"Phew! It's good to know that he is tied-up." Garden peas said with a sigh of relief.

"I know. We are safe." Mrs. Lady Finger heaved a similar sigh of relief.

"Let's go and see what has happened?" Nerdy Spinach Leaf suggested curiously.

Others all nodded except Wise Bitter- Gourd, "I am sensing something fishy. I think we should be very careful." Bitter-Gourd warned.

They all walked towards the tied-up phagocyte. Two ropes were fastened against his stomach and he was tied up against the wall. He looked at them angrily.

"You are back. You trespassers! How dare you come back?" He snarled at them.

"Who tied you up?" Chubby Cauliflower asked cautiously from a distance, afraid he would loosen himself up and eat his leaves again.

"Other trespassers like you who don't belong in lungs." He told them furiously. "I patrol this lobby. And I will eat trespassers like you all."

"Yeah we got that! But can you please give us the name of other trespassers?" Nerdy Spinach Leaf urged.

"We did." The previous Loaf of Breads, who were guarding the entrance of brain stood behind them.

All the vegetables looked at each other in terror. They took a long breath and sprinted towards the staircase. But before they could climb down more than three steps, a huge rope was thrown on them. Tight knots were tied up at their waist. They were all tied up together.

The other end of rope was in hand of the bread. They laughed on them. "Obviously it was us. Who else did you think?" The brown bread told them cheekily.

"And look down the stairs. We have tied up every nutrient in the lungs," and true to his words when vegetables looked down they saw all the nutrients like white and red cells were tied up to the pole. They could also see bubbles of air being tied up.

"You hijacked the station!" Nerdy Spinach Leaf asked unbelievably.

"Not just station! Even the trains!" White loaf said proudly. "Our loaf driver now drives the train."

All vegetables stared at them furiously.

"And yes before I forget. Let me add that we are also very proud..." White bread started but before he could finish Brown bread pushed him away.

"No let me tell them." The brown bread insisted.

"Don't be a fool. I started it. Let me speak it." The white bread argued back.

"I will speak it." The brown Bread declared and they both started quarrelling amongst themselves. They started pushing each other now.

The vegetables rolled their eyes at their immature behaviour. "Somebody please tell us what else have you all done?" Nerdy Spinach Leaf prayed to an invisible god.

"We have even hijacked the entire small intestine." The white bread broke it proudly.

The face of vegetables fell in shock.

"And kidnapped each of your armies." The brown bread added in enthusiastically.

"We have captured them in the Toilet jail and we will churn them in urine. Then we will flush them out of the body. " They both said delighted at once.

All The vegetables lost the colour of their face. They all looked shocked.

"Even my son?" Mrs Lady Finger asked with tears springing in her eyes.

"Yes, even your son." White loaf told her casually, "Hence, I suggest you all to come with us back to brain. If you all co-operate then we will leave the intestine alone."

All the vegetables nodded their heads sadly, having no other option. The loaf of breads smiled at each other. The vegetables had bought their story. Otherwise it would have been very difficult to bring them to the brain without a struggle. Now they will come with them quietly, and when the vegetable army in intestine would get to know that their leaders have been captured, they would surrender the entire intestine for exchange of their leader. And soon small intestine would be theirs. Breads were all too smart!

They pushed the tied-up bunch of vegetables on the platform towards the train. Once inside the train the vegetables saw that the other nutrients in the train were tied-up to poles too. They all looked sad and gloomy. Breads dragged them towards a seat and instructed them to sit down. Vegetables did that without complain, since they had no option but to listen to whatever loafs of bread told them; at least for the sake of their armies and family.

Train started. But Instead of going in direction of the brain it started moving in opposite direction.

"Lord help me! He is again driving in opposite direction." White loaf let out his breath in frustration.

"Yes he is again going south instead of north." Brown Bread nodded his head in disappointment. "Wait. I will go and give him a piece of my mind." He said and disappeared in another chamber of train.

All nutrients looked sadly at the vegetables. The vegetables looked back at them with an equally sad gaze.

Suddenly the train started moving on the white strips instead of moving inside the white strips. The train started spiralling round-round on those strips like a merry-go-round ride.

"Oh Lord! He is driving on the Ribs." The white Loaf face-palmed himself. "He really has no brain."

"Tell him to drive inside the ribs not on it." He shouted in the compartment where Brown Bread had just disappeared. The train started moving erratically on the narrow white strips of the ribs. Many a times it was going to fall down from the stripes but the driver loaf pulled it back on the stripes. The White Bread had to clutch on the pole of train to avoid falling down.

"This is not the route, on top of it he is driving on narrow ribs, on top of it, he is arguing with me." The Brown Bread shouted as he busted back in the room. Even he held on heavily to a pole to avoid losing his balance.

Suddenly the lights in the train started fluctuating. A grumbling sound echoed in the whole body. One by one each light became dim before it eventually became dark. Both the loaf of breads huffed in annoyance. Brown bread left the pole he was clutching to and walked up to the switch board. The train was circling from one strip to another with a rash speed. Many-a-times Brown Bread lost his footing and fell down. He finally reached the board. He flipped the switch up and down but the lights did not come back.

Suddenly the whole train derailed and fell down from the rib strip. It took a few tumbles and finally crashed against the bottom of the ribs

There was a complete darkness in the train. All the vegetables which were tied-up together shifted here and there. If and when one would shift, their common rope would make other shift too, and right now lemon was shifting a lot much to the irritation of other vegetables. He was also leaking lot of puss which was burning other vegetables skin.

Suddenly a bunch of fruits wearing neon mask entered the train chambers. Calcium knives were in their hands. They quickly started ripping the ropes of every nutrient and pushed those nutrients in their bag. One of them walked up to the vegetables and tore apart their ropes too. He then tried to push those vegetables in their bag. But the vegetables pushed that fruit away. That fruit then proceeded to the next batch of nutrients on the opposite seat. Their neon mask was the only source of light in the darkness.

"Hey!" White bread screamed at fruit and pulled out his own calcium knife. But before he could attack the neon mask wearing fruit, the fruit himself attacked the white bread. White crumbs of bread started falling on ground. The vegetables opened their mouths in shock. They had just witnessed a murder in front of them. A murder of bread!

That neon masked fruit was quickly shoving the nutrients in his bag when the brown bread attacked him from the back. He striked his knife right into his back. A river of Juice started flowing out of his body. Another Neon mask wearing fruit attacked brown bread from behind and shredded him to crumbs.

All the vegetables gasped.

It was a blood bath! Miss Lady Leek clutched her heart.

Sensing an opportunity they quickly got up from their seat and moved towards the door. In darkness they bumped and fell into various things. But they somehow managed to reach the doors of train and quickly opened it. They moved out of it. It was all darkness outside the train too. The train lay there derailed. They hastily moved around the derailed train and started walking in an uncertain direction. They caught each other's hands. That helped them to walk miles without tripping in darkness.

"I think the body has become unconscious," the wise Bitter-Gourd concluded.

"Hence this darkness...!" Nerdy Spinach Leaf agreed with him.

They walked for minutes and minutes in darkness before they finally saw some light in distance.

Chapter 18

War.

The light in the distance was blinding. The more steps they took the darkness was switching into light. Soon they reached the lighted area. There was a river right in front of their eyes, and on that river was a beautiful bridge.

Oxygen bubbles were floating in the air. Few of them busted right in front of Miss Lady Leek's face. She enjoyed the coolness of it.

"Oxy Facials are so costly now-a-days. These are far better than them", she whispered delightfully to Mrs. Lady Finger, who just shrugged, "I wouldn't know, I have never done them."

"I have done plenty. I was bought by beautician before in auction. Her refrigerator had oxygen filtered air. Once I heard her saying to her neighbour, that it keeps our skin nice."

"Seems fancy."

"Oh! It was. I loved her a lot, until one day; she decided to add juice of a person close to me in her face pack. She bleeded a lot of juice that day and died." Miss Lady Leek said remembering the kind Lady Fig who was like her mother.

"Oh it sounds harsh."

"Yes it was horrific. Her juice was dripping all over the refrigerator shelf." She had tears in her eyes now.

"So how does this facial work?" Mrs. Lady Finger asked quickly trying to change the subject.

"Just let the bubbles burst on your face."

As they walked down the river, the entire bank of the river was carpented with yellow, pink, red, white and green flowers till the eyes could see, making it look very pretty.

"Wow! Look at all these flowers!" Mrs. Lady Finger said excitedly.

They could hear pounding sounds of liquid from a distance. Three sparkling waterfalls were thundering down the stones at the bottom of the river.

The vegetables were quite disturbed seeing the waterfalls, since the whole body was in drought. But what really angered them the most was the glorious blood falls besides the waterfall.

"This blood falls are boiling my blood." Lemon said pissed. "The whole body is unconscious and this place is sparkling with water and blood waterfalls. What a slap on our face?" Lemon spoke angrily.

"It's those fruits. They are decoiting trains and stealing nutrients." Nerdy Spinach Leaf spoke after a thought. "They should be imprisoned in the Toilet jail."

"That blood looks so refreshingly divine. It could do wonders for the body. Too bad they wasted it by turning it into a blood-fall." Mrs. Lady Finger said disappointedly.

"They are so selfish. They are thieves. They have robbed the body of their nutrition." Ms Miss Lady Leek spoke bitterly

"This is evil." Chubby Cauliflower spitted.

****

On the other end of the bridge, the Apple caught a glimpse of their nightmare approaching them. He cursed under his breath. He was waiting for young fruits, who would return with the loot they would loot.

He gave out a sweet smile when he saw the vegetables crossing the bridge and coming closer to him.

"Welcome to our humble aboard. What brings you here?" Apple said over-sugary, while greeting them. "Well not that humble but nevertheless."

"We were in the train that was just got decoited." Lemon said cheekily.

"Oh that's a shame." Apple said quickly, looking down uncomfortably.

"Where are we exactly?" Chubby Cauliflower asked curiously.

"You are in the liver. The new beautiful organ of the body." Apple said proudly.

"Good to see you fruits have done really well for yourself," wise Bitter-Guard faked sweetly, putting his hands around the apple's shoulders.

"We try," Apple smiled awkwardly.

Soon they were approaching a beautiful three storey house as they walked deeper towards a clearing on which the house stood.

"You should come inside our humble house; others would be excited to meet you." Apple offered quickly, trying to change the topic. The pleasing house was made from exotic wooden sticks. It had beautiful windows with drapes made of leaves. A beautiful veil of grape ran around the house artfully. The walls of the house were coloured in pink food colour. It had statues of orange, apple, banana, grapes and the members of berry family like raspberry, cranberry and Strawberry carved on it.

A huge statue of fruit basket stood in front of the house.

"That's a tribute to all the fruits living in the house." Apple informed gesturing towards the statue.

"Lovely! That's such a sweet thing to do." Chubby Cauliflower taunted giving a bright forced smile.

As they stepped on the porch, their footsteps could be heard inside the living room where everyone in the house had gathered, waiting impatiently for the loot to arrive, in affair to sort them out.

While an Orange was rolled up on an arm chair, the berry family took the couch. The bunch of grapes preferred cosying up in their bowl placed on the coffee table. Banana fancied leaning against the couch so that he could flirt with the strawberry. A tomato was also sitting somewhere in the same living room waiting for his child.

An elderly apple stomped his feet impatiently against his rug. His ears perked up at the sound and without really glancing thoroughly, he announced,

"Oh thank almighty!" he spoke throwing his hands up, "They are finally here with the loot." But as soon as he saw his visitors he bit back his tongue.

"Hmm…..oh no not them!" Cranberry spoke indifferently. She was a bit disappointed to see her black nail paint chipping off. She will have to re-apply immediately. She even hated how dark red her body was. She always fancied a black body like grapes which would suit her gothic moods and needs. Meanwhile the black grapes always fancied to have the pink blush of raspberry.

Orange narrowed her eyes and looked bitterly towards the strawberry, who was wrapped up in flirting with her crush banana.

"Sorry! We don't have your loot!" Chubby Cauliflower apologized sassily.

"Hmm..that's okay." The elder apple uttered stunned. "Well, welcome to our house. Surprised to see you visiting us," He spoke shaking himself out of the shock.

Apple tried to catch elder apple's eyes to warn him against bringing up that subject but he failed and elder apple kept on speaking, "So what brings you here?"

"We were in the train that was just got decoited." Chubby Cauliflower spoke sassily again.

"Oh that's a pity! By whom?" Elder Apple inquired with full honesty.

Apple face palmed himself. Today was not a day for him to be so dumb. "By nobody," He said loudly to elderly Apple.

"By a bunch of fruits, Some tomato, apple, banana, raspberry and cranberry to be precise." The vegetables suddenly yelled at all the fruits in living room.

"Don't scream on me. That's their kids." Strawberry expressed annoyed. "I don't have kids," she pouted, "not yet" she added after she glimpsed at banana.

"Ours would have joined dacoity too if they weren't so lazy. They are still sleeping upstairs." One of the grape in bunches of Grape spoke, defeated and tired. "A mother tries and tries, but if the kid refuses to listen what can…" She started crying.

"Okay enough with your sob story." Apple junior cropped her mid-way. "And yes we did it. It was our kids who decoited the train." He admitted it without a tinge of regret in his voice.

"You must be such proud parents, raising your kids to be dacoits." The vegetables taunted.

"They are just earning their bread and butter." Strawberry replied flipping them off.

"King bread would be so pleased to hear it that idiom." Miss Lady Leek threw shade on her bitterly.

"When we came here first this place looked like a bloated Tomato." Elder Apple informed the vegetables. Tomato looked up at him.

"Sorry tomato. I didn't mean it." The elder apple apologised when he realised his mistake and then turned his attention back to vegetables.

"Like I was saying this place was like a bloated tomato. We made it healthy and a beautiful place again." Elder apple continued.

"We transferred this place in to the heaven, it looks now." Cranberry added in proudly.

"At the cost of body?" spinach asked unbelievably.

"Excuse me?" Apple asked offended, "Liver is part of body too."

"Precisely! Nobody notices when liver is suffering. Body can die if something happens to Liver." Cranberry added in angrily.

"That was your duty to do it and so you did it." Wise Bitter-Gourd stated. "But now liver is healthy so release all the extra blood that you have. We want the blood from blood-fall."

"We formed that blood from the Beetroots. They had come to know that we are in liver. So they came to liver. They said they missed tomatoes and had come to visit them. When we told them about the difficulty in liver, they were more than ready to sacrifice themselves for betterment of liver." Apple Junior informed the vegetables. "They are true patriotics."

All vegetables were shocked. They had been travelling all over the body for Beetroots while beetroots had been in liver all this while. They were relieved, but shocked and angry at the same time. Relieved, that their search finally ended, shocked at the new piece of information, and angry that they were kept in dark, all this time.

"All of them?" Nerdy Spinach Leaf asked shocked.

"Yes all of them."

"So?" Lemon raised his eyebrow curiously.

"So we used the required amount of blood and that blood fall is extra blood for maintenance and future use."

"Well body kind of required blood right n..." Mrs. Lady Finger started.

"Oh! And now we have also signalled the brain, with permission from king bread, that all the beetroots will be henceforth transferred over here directly!" Apple said cutting Mrs. Lady Finger in.

"So that means you want to have all Beetroots for yourself, and nothing for the body." Mrs. Lady Finger asked shocked at their shamelessness.

"Well you can always have other food to form your own blood supply." Apple suggested calmly.

"Right now the body is doomed."

"It's not like the girl is eating anything much healthy now. This is all that the body has and if this finishes too, how would it get re-filled? The body was doomed anyways." Cranberry said rejecting their offer to take the blood.

"The whole body has switched off. Everything is dark because the girl is unconscious. We need your extra blood." Vegetables argued back desperately.

"We don't wish the body good as well as bad. We are merely in the state of indifference." Apple junior spoke casually, "Sorry we can't give our extra-blood to you."

"But this is your home too. If the body is destroyed, where will you go? You will be destroyed too." Mrs. Lady Finger threw a final brick at vegetables.

That shut them up good.

****

Footsteps could be heard again on the porch. Voices talking urgently could be heard from outside. There was a fear in their voice. Doors opened and five young fruits entered inside the house.

Now that the vegetables were seeing them carefully, they really were very young!

The young tomato had held the body of young apple in his arms.

Apple junior's and Apple senior's breath got stuck seeing the dead body of young apple. They were struck with tragedy. Tears streamed down their face and they broke down. Every fruit gathered around to console them.

Young Cranberry went running to his mommy and shouted something to her, "Mommy mommy! Quick they are coming! Quickly pack your bags. Or else they will slice us with their knives." Junior cranberry told her mom with wide frantic eyes. "They even have bigger earthworms than us. They will eat us in one bite!"

"What are you talking about?" Cranberry asked him disinterested.

Young Cranberry looked at young Tomato.

"Remember you told us that if we don't go to sleep early, king bread will come and steal our seeds?" young Tomato spoke to his dad after he handed over the body of young apple to his father.

"Ahh...yeah?" Master Tomato raised his eyes.

"Well I might have gone to bed late yesterday!" young tomato said ashamed, "and now they are coming to steal our seeds."

"Our lineage ends here. We were going so well as grandfather, father and son. But now you are gone and here I was dreaming about great-grand child." Senior Apple sobbed heavily.

"Who told you that?" Cranberry inquired clearly un-amused by her kid's whining.

"Young Tomato." Young Cranberry pointed towards the young tomato. They all looked towards the young tomato, who was talking hush-hush in his dad's ears.

"I told you not to scare your kid too much like this. Now he is going crazy." Cranberry rolled her eyes.

"He is not. They raised white flag at the border of the liver." Master Tomato spoke. Young Tomato was clearly the eldest of the younger lot and led the younger pack.

"Is that true?" Cranberry asked Young Cranberry, who had extremely purple cheeks.

"Yes, I saw a white loaf hoisting the flag outside the liver border, myself." Young Cranberry spoke sincerely whatever he saw. "It has poster size photo of King Bread on it."

Cranberry became purpler after hearing that. She was furious.

"It's all because of these stupid vegetables. Breads have followed them here." Cranberry spoke fiercely.

"White Flag means war. White symbolises King Bread domination. Every organ ruled by bread has a white flag hoisted outside its entrance. Apart from liver all areas have a white flag hoisted. Sadly now a bright white flag stands on entrance of our liver. And it's all because of this vegetables." Strawberry spoke angrily.

"Precisely! White means war!" Young Cranberry spoke confidently. "This is what Master Tomato had taught us in study section."

Master Tomato beamed proudly.

"But sadly he is confused about his own race. He doesn't even know whether his ancestors were fruits or vegetables." Miss Lady Leek taunted.

Mrs Lady Finger looked at Leek disappointedly. What she said was rude.

"Miss Lady Leek, I had my identity crisis. I never felt like a vegetable. I felt out of the place. But over here between all my fellow fruits I feel at home. My confusion is a thing of past. I am finally home." Tomato spoke calmly and maturely.

"And stop pointing fingers at Tomato." Cranberry spoke defensively, "We have protected liver so far. We are not fools to roam around the body on tour leaving over area exposed. But look at what you have done. You have let them take your kingdom and now you have attracted them over here. They followed you over here. Now we will have a war." she scolded them.

All the vegetables kept quiet. They did agree with her point; so how were they supposed to argue back? Even the weeping apples in corner looked at them as if their son's death was their fault.

"King Bread will be marching here soon with his army. But knowing how heavy, out of shape and lazy they are, it will take them double time to reach here." Nerdy Spinach Leaf spoke trying to save themselves from all the accusation.

"Yes! They might be huge in number but they are pretty dumb." Chubby Cauliflower nodded along with spinach.

"That gives us plenty of time to gather our worms from their bills. Pull out fresh fungi from the refrigerator and also sharpen our calcium knives to cut breads to pieces." Apples ranted determined to take their revenge from breads.

"We will build a stone wall on bridge and have our armies stationed there." Cranberry added.

"We have no time to waste then. We have to be quick on our feet. We will have one third of our armies stationed at the murder hole on the terrace of the house." Tomato explained hastily to other ,"they will stand behind the hole and fire things like rocks all coated in boiling oil from it to fry them as soon as the approach us. We will…"

"Excuse me I am sorry to interrupt your defence jamming section." Nerdy Spinach Leaf started sheepishly. "But we need to take that extra blood to intestine to revive the body."

"That extra blood is ours. We refuse to give it." Cranberry said stubbornly.

"That blood is not yours. You are a thief." Ms Miss Lady Leek said equally threateningly.

"And after the war we will require it the most." Cranberry argued.

"The body requires it now." Leek argued back.

"Our army will fight with full braveness today while your army in toilet jail are preparing themselves to be flushed out of the body." Cranberry spoke like an evil monster.

Miss Lady Leek was taken aback by her harsh words. But she did not show it on her face.

"Once the war gets over, the body will be dead, were will you go then?" Miss Lady Leek asked judgingly.

"We will survive!" Cranberry said confidently.

Both Cranberry and Miss Lady Leek stared at each other furiously, fumes coming out of their nostrils and their faces barely inches from each other. Everybody stood silently watching them until Tomato screamed, "Time to prepare."

All fruits started panicking. Chaos erupted as they started running here and there.

"Will you support us?" Tomato asked Wise Bitter-Gourd considering he was the wisest amongst them.

"For now yes, only because they are our common enemy," Bitter Gourd answered back maturely.

And they shook hands.

Refrigerator was opened in the kitchen and young fruit kids carried huge crates of fungus and placed them on the table one by one. The chill from the refrigerator numbed their hands. It reminded them of the days they were imported from Australia in refrigerators to keep them fresh. They removed the fresh fungus packed in the crates and silently hoped they would be enough to infect the entire army of bread.

Heaps of long and fat earthworms were being pulled out from their bills and kept on tables. They slithered and hissed sharply. They hated being brought out of their bills.

Huge insect trap nets were built outside the house to capture enemies' insects. All the parents applied insect repellents to their kids before slathering on few themselves.

"It's like sunscreen. You should always use them." Grapes said as she handed over the bottle to the vegetables after she was done coating her kids.

Armies were rounded up from their huts and were gathered. They too applied insect repellents, so that it would be difficult for opposite party's insects to eat them.

Few fruit army immediately got to the work of sharpening their calcium knives. A shredder machine was stolen by tomato before entering the body from the kitchen of the person who had bought him from the market. He had stolen it so that he could escape from being shredded. He had also stolen kitchen knives so that he wouldn't be cut open. He distributed those knives amongst the armies.

The first batch of army was dispatched to stand on murder hole on terrace.

****

Five hours went by, as fruit army along with protectors stood by the bridge restlessly waiting for signs of enemy approaching it. It was hard to figure out what time of day it would be, as skin had stopped sun rays penetrating through it. But usually this would be the time when Sun would settle down and dusk would grow fast. The setting sun would glitter a hard orange colour on the tips of their knives. But right now it was a gloomy darkness all around. Many of the soldiers were busy erecting the stone wall on bridge behind them. It was almost complete.

"Apple! Leader! Do you see this?" Banana shivered as he pointed towards the opposite side of the river.

"I would say they are rather hard to miss." Apple junior pointed out as he studied hundreds of bread loafs approaching the bridge. They were much more than what he had anticipated. Gigantic to be precise. He was not so sure about fighting the war now. His army was too few to tackle such a huge number. He let his gaze wander amongst all the sea of breads. In middle of that sea was an old aged bread wearing an orange cape. He was carried in a basket by few of his bodyguards. Apple junior's eyes hovered over on an ocean of cars at the back, each holding different kind of weapons like calcium and kitchen knives, Spoons, Juice processors, blenders and shredders. They looked fully equipped to remove all the juice from his armies.

He asked one of his Apple soldier to come forward and whispered in his ears. The soldier nodded and turned back. He walked amidst the fruit army and disappeared somewhere only to come back with a green flag. The other fruits gaped in surprise as they watched Apple Junior take the flag from the soldier and stepped forward from his position. He perched the green flag in the ground.

From the distance, through a glass window in the house the vegetables were clearly observing their every move. Their face lost colour as soon as the saw the apple perch the green flag in the ground. A mixture of fear and anger seeded through them.

"What? They surrendered already." Mrs. Lady Finger gaped in surprise.

"Traitors! We should have never trusted them." Miss Lady Leek muttered in her breath. "They were always a bunch of cowards." Chubby Cauliflower groaned.

"First lazy to do their work, then thieves, and now cowards. I wonder what next surprise they will spring on us." Lemon spitted while Garden peas and Wise Bitter-Gourd shook their heads in disappointment.

"Green Flag also means to talk." Nerdy Spinach Leaf announced, "They might want to negotiate instead of fighting the war."

"What are they going to talk about?" Mrs. Lady Finger asked scared.

"They are going to sell us." Nerdy Spinach Leaf stated bitterly. Lady Finger shivered. Outside their room they could hear loud footsteps approaching their room and stopping at their door. Below their window, few fruit soldiers paced towards their side of wall to prevent the vegetables from escaping from the window.

"And now we are trapped!" They all exclaimed at once.

"Again," Mrs Lady Finger cried.

****

Simultaneously, a green flag was waved from the enemies' side. A soldier came forward from the bread army. Apple being the first to wave the flag took two steps forward as he saw a soldier approaching him across the bridge. The bread soldier escorted apple to king bread.

As soon as they crossed the bridge, they entered an ocean of bread soldiers as far as the sight could go, all stepping aside to let the Apple be escorted to the king bread. They were lazy and slow in their movement. It took them so much time to move aside. Pity they were in huge number or else his fruit army would have defeated them in a moment.

Now they were fast approaching the cape wearing King Bread seated in a basket held by a bunch of bread body-guard. He was smirking and smiling evilly as he looked over at the apple approaching his basket. He gestured his bodyguard to put him down. He got up from his place and stepped outside his basket.

"Why the talk? Do you surrender already?" He asked proudly.

"No. But I have a better proposition, since you see; we are not ones who are really the enemies?

"O! But we are enemies. We are supposed to destroy you right now." Bread laughed airily.

"Or it could easily be the other way around." Apple stood its ground.

The caped king let out an impulsive snort on hearing that.

"I like your confidence even though you have very few soldiers to boost of." Bread appraised.

"Anyways why cause destruction to each other, when we have a common enemy." Apple suggested smartly.

Bread raised his eyebrow in surprise, not believing a word he just heard.

"Are you implying the vegetables?" The king asked.

"Yes! The very same."

"But I thought vegetables and fruits have an eternal bond to save body from all kind of troubles."

"Well! At least not in this body." Apple rolled his eyes, "We hate them with as much angst as you do. They are irritating and nagging. They suck all the joy out of living."

"Like a juicer!" Bread fostered.

"Just like a juicer." Apple huffed in affirmation.

"I don't really require you. Small Intestine is already under our control." Bread proclaimed boldly.

"Oh! Is it really now?" Apple asked dubiously. "Stop playing me a fool! You definitely attacked intestine but sadly you got attacked instead. Their vegetable army destroyed your bread army in minutes. They are mighty and too strong to be destroyed."

King Bread looked at him in shock. He had all the inside information.

"You don't know our strength!" Bread argued.

"We both know you will need us to take control on small intestine."

"Fine!" Bread caved in; "I think!" he shrugged. "But how do I trust you?"

"Because we have held vegetable leaders as captive. We will hand over to you at the time when usually the first ray of light breaks through the skin."

"No. You hand them to me by the time it's usually very late night."

Apple thought for a minute. He looked over the sea of brad soldiers.

"Can't do." He started shaking his head, "Unless you need ask half of your soldiers to go back to brains."

The king thought for a few moments before eventually caving in.

"Deal."

"Deal."

****

Apple stood on the bridge, at time when it's usually late night. He was overlooking the view of their then enemies-now-friends partners. Piles of tents were rooted in the ground. Many pumpkin shell cars were parked at a distance. Few tents lay abandoned. It was clear from number of tents that lay abandoned that half of the bread soldiers had gone back to brain. Now that he had witnessed the situation first hand, he was sure he had played the breads fool successfully. His slimmer doubts had melted. Now that they were few in number he and his army had chances of destroying them. Even though it was an established fact that Breads were lazy and would grab a freeway with a tight fist, still a knot of suspicion tugged in the heart of Apple. Apple promised King Bread that fruits will help him to take control on intestine. But he also knew King Bread wanted body domination. After capturing intestine only liver would be left as King Bread already dominated all other body parts. He would spare no expense in destroying fruits to get control on liver. Hence it was important to destroy breads. Besides this body was their home too where would they go if this body dies?

But mostly importantly a Bread soldier had killed his son. There was a fire in his eyes and a desire to take revenge of his son's death. Now he will burn them to a toast.

****

There was a quick and secretive activities going on behind in the three storey bungalow, just diagonal to where apple was standing. The entire vegetable team were busy going in-and-out of the rooms to select the best window to jump from on the second storey of bungalow. They wanted to determine the best route of escape from all the multi-storey windows on the second floor.

"This one seems slippery".

"That one is slanting."

"This one's roof is too low. It will hit us on our head. "

They came out of the last room dejected. Mrs Lady Finger was carrying three jugs of blood which fruits eventually gave her to save the body. All fruit protectors were currently somewhere outside the house, roaming around the breads to burn them. They were so scared fruits would give them up to save themselves, but seems like they had a change of heart. Took them time, but better late than never. All young baby fruits were currently packed up in their beds to sleep. Except a baby tomato, who was watching them secretly from behind a wall near the staircase.

They had no choice but to pick a least horrible window from the all the windows, on the second storey. The windows on first storey were battle-field facing and would make their escaping noticeable to bread. They assumed third storey windows would be too high. They would Jump themselves to death from there. They decided the window of last room on second floor they exited would be it, as it was better than the other room's windows. They again entered the last room. They pushed the curtains aside and once again unlocked the window. Lemon being the shortest amongst them decided to try first. But the roof of that window was too low. He had to squeeze himself a bit lower. Drops of puss started leaking from his body as he pressed his body too hard to fit himself on the window still.

"I have a secret place." Young tomato said shyly from behind. Some of the vegetables turned their heads in surprise to see a young, shy looking tomato, fidgeting with his hands, looking awkwardly at them.

"Oh sweetie! Even I had a secret place when I was your age. I used hide in drawers of the kitchen. Nobody would ever find me there. It was perfect spot for hide and seek." Mrs Lady Finger said sweetly. She could see her son in him.

"I used to hide in my hiding spot because all the other kids would pluck my leaves." Chubby Cauliflower said recalling his nightmare.

"You would like to see mine?" Young tomato asked chubby Cauliflower shyly.

"That's wonderfully but we don't really have time to see your secret place." Miss Lady Leek announced as she tried to shoo away the child.

"I jump from there all the time." He said innocently to Miss Lady Leek.

Lemon finally was able to fit himself through the window and then he jumped from it. He collided with the ground with a "plop" sound.

Other vegetables suddenly turned towards the child tomato attentively.

"Really! Jump! Would you like to show us the place?" Ms Miss Lady Leek said, suddenly extremely sweetly now.

Baby Tomato perked up with excitement. "Yes! Yes. Nobody ever comes over there to play with me because I am the youngest."

Baby Tomato then looked hopefully at Ms Miss Lady Leek, "but will you play with me?"

Miss Lady Leek faked a big sweet smile and nodded.

"If everybody knows about your secret place then how come it's your secret place?" Mrs Lady Finger teased him playfully. Baby tomato looked at her confusingly.

Baby Tomato tugged at Miss Lady Leek's hand as he wanted to take her up the staircase to his hiding place. Miss Lady Leek looked behind at the other vegetables doubtfully. They just shrugged. They all started climbing the staircase to the third storey.

The end of staircase opened up to a space below the dark roof of the house. A light of beam shone through a small window at the end of the room. A small supporting plank was attached to the window from outside. It also wasn't battle-field facing. Nobody from bread army would sight them from far-far away while escaping. It was perfect for jumping.

It had no slanting or sloppy window panes nor did it have any low canopy hanging to hit them in the head. Beautiful leave veils were running outside the window. But their biggest advantage would be the wooden steps attached to the bark of tomato tree near the window.

"That's where I come from!" Baby Tomato told them in his baby voice pointing towards the tree. "I come here often to meet my baby sisters and brothers who are not yet ripe to be plucked. And sometimes..." He blushed while talking about the incident.

"Yes go on." Mrs Lady Finger encouraged him "I and baby strawberry use this attic window to sneak away for a stroll in the farms at nights."

"They have farms too?" Miss Lady Leek asked Nerdy Spinach Leaf a bit taken aback.

"Probably." Spinach shrugged.

"Did you attach those wooden steps yourself?" Mrs Lady Finger asked, still chit-chatting with the little boy.

"Oh no! That's done by the grandpa, when my siblings ripe, they just climb down the stairs and enter the house." Young tomato squeaked. "Sadly my grandpa has perished now. But he left his seeds behind! I will get it for you." He jumped excitedly and went to his bed to get the seeds.

"All right! Enough chit-chatting let's get back to the business! I will fly to the wooden stairs first and then climb them down." Nerdy Spinach Leaf Clapped to get everybody's attention.

"Why don't you fly till the bottom ground? You are just a leaf." Miss Lady Leek Suggested.

"It's too high from here. I don't want to die." He said with an obvious face.

"Okay." Miss Lady Leek rolled her eyes.

Spinach just shrugged and flew out of the window and before they could even blink he was balancing his thin legs on the wooden piece and had climbed down the stairs.

"Wow that was fast!" Chubby Cauliflower murmured under his breath before tumbling out of the window himself and rolling down the supporting plank before reaching the end of it. He jumped the distance between the plank and stairs and landed on the tree stairs. Even he bounced down the stairs effortlessly.

Bitter-Gourd and Miss Lady Leek followed his action by walking towards the end of the plank, jumping the distance and climbing down the wooden stairs and joining the others below. But unlike spinach, Bitter-Gourd had difficulty balancing his thin legs on the wooden stairs. Mrs Lady Finger though, asked by others to carry the jugs of blood, refused to give its responsibility to others. She skilfully balanced the three jugs in her hand and climbed down the stairs like a ballerina.

Then all the vegetables walked the grounds towards the garage in the backyard. They all looked towards the Pumpkin car and then at each other. Finally they all got in the car except Miss Lady Leek.

"I am not getting into this oxygen-eating-carbon dioxide-releasing monster." Miss Lady Leek scrunched up her face in disgust.

"Just get in." Lemon ordered her.

Miss Lady Leek huffed and got in the five-seater pumpkin car.

"I prefer Orange and Watermelon carrier over Pumpkin. Even-though they are smaller than pumpkin shell as they are more oxygen efficient vehicles." She kept ranting in the car throughout the way.

The pumpkin car was driven by the Nerdy Spinach Leaf. Besides him was Bitter-Gourd and all the other vegetables were crammed in backseat.

Nerdy Spinach looked ahead at the road. Wise Bitter-Gourd was instructing the direction of the road from besides. Lemon at back was staring at Miss Lady Leek, who was busy looking distastefully at all smoke created by their Pumpkin car.

Chubby Cauliflower had gone to sleep. Journeys always made him sleepy. Peas were talking amongst themselves in their pod. While Mrs Lady Finger held all the three jugs of blood tightly to her chest. She also covered the top of jugs by her other hand to avoid any spillage on the bumpy ride.

The carrier kept shaking over dead cells, boils and random hair. They journeyed over kidney and pancreas. While Pancreas had dried up, kidneys had an odour of urine in air. The whole body was in absolute darkness.

'Thankfully nobody is following us', Lemon thought. Probably he thought too soon, as he sighted a minor movement from corner from his eyes. He sensed somebody was watching their car. Someone was following them from the corner of his eyes. They had almost reached small intestine. They had to be careful now that the whole small intestine was under breads control.

"There are Bread loafs patrolling the area." lemon informed the others in the car.

"Gods above! O almighty! We better be careful then." Miss Lady Leek expressed her fear quite dramatically.

"Yes we have to stay cautious. Nobody wants to end up in Memory loss chamber again." Lemon agreed with her.

"Run the car below the shadows of tree," wise Bitter-Gourd suggested.

Spinach vroomed the car more towards the corner of the road below the trees."

"Though I have to say, I have learnt and grown so much." Chubby Cauliflower suddenly spoke emotionally after waking from his sleep.

"Yes we appreciate the importance of our job more. I would happily sacrifice myself now rather than just seeing it as a duty." Nerdy Spinach Leaf Spoke like an enlightened soul.

"Well! It's good to leave as a martyr rather than just perish." Lemon agreed whole-heartedly.

"I am just worried about my son. He can't even walk and talk properly yet. How can such a small child be held in jail?" Mrs. Lady Finger sobbed.

"Well many things are beyond everybody's mind." Chubby Cauliflower consoled her.

Lady Finger held the jugs of blood more tightly to her chest now. Their mission would be successful when they would successfully offload the blood on digestion track. From Digestion track they would automatically carried to different parts of body and the girl would wake up.

"Our main priority right now is not to get caught before we can offload the jugs of blood in the digestion." Nerdy Spinach Leaf spoke on an urgent note. "We can get caught after that. But at least the body can wake up again."

There was crunching noises in the bushes. A set of Pumpkin cars appeared behind them. They were being followed.

"Those bunches of loafers are right behind us. Run, run." Lemon shouted in ears of Spinach.

"Don't run. Fly"

"Loose them"

Lemon kept screaming.

"But how?" Spinach panicked and pressed the accelerator button and increased the speed of car."

"Remember our mantra: - Do not get caught before we eject the blood in the digestion. I repeat do not get caught before we eject blood in the digestion." Lemon told spinach sternly.

"Stop scarring him. He is driving. He will create an accident." Miss Lady Leek said deadpanned eyeing Lemon threateningly. But Lemon was still very jumpy. He kept looking back at the other pumpkin cars. They were still hot on their heels.

"We have almost reached small intestine. A little bit more gas and we will reach digestion." Bitter-Gourd spoke calmly.

Spinach hit the pedal some more and gas started running over the limit. They started losing them.

"Fly! Fly! Fly." Chubby Cauliflower screamed and screeched from behind.

And very soon the cars following them were out of sight. They all heaved a sigh of relief. But soon they saw an orange and yellow carrier from front coming towards them with full gusto.

"Turn back!"

"Turn back you idiot!" Lemon barked orders in spinach's ears from back.

"Please sit down." Miss Lady Leek said irritated as she pulled Lemon back to his seat.

"Don't take U-turn. Those previous cars following us will corner us." Bitter-Gourd suggested spinach, but it was too late as he had already u-turned the carrier. Soon true to words of Bitter-Gourd they could see those previous pumpkin cars at a distance. Spinach turned his car left in a small alley.

He parked the Pumpkin carrier on the sides of the alley hoping their followers wouldn't be able to spot them in the darkness. After a lapse of almost an hour and no sight of any other yellow and orange carrier apart from theirs Spinach decided to turn on the car around. They were now moving on the intestine roads cautiously, keeping an alert eye for their predators. Mrs Lady Finger tightly clenched the jugs in her fist. Nothing should happen to them or otherwise the purpose of their whole trip would flow in gutters.

They were approaching digestion at eye blinking speed. They were just fifteen paces away from digestion, when they spotted the former two pumpkin cars hot on their tails again.

"No matter what happens, just throw the blood in digestion," Chubby Cauliflower urged Mrs Lady Finger, who nodded her head seriously.

They were just five paces away when a large stone was hurdled towards the wheels of their car. Their whole pumpkin car turned upside-down and fell on its side. All the vegetables in the car were thrown out of the car. Mrs Lady Finger held the jugs tightly even when falling. She was determined to avoid the spillage of blood from any of the three jugs. She covered their tops tightly with her palms to avoid any of their spillage. She quickly got up and ran towards the digestion and threw the blood on the tract before her predators could attack her. Various noises started erupting from Digestion. Those noises were an indicator that the blood has been accepted.

All the vegetables heaved a sigh of relief.

"Ahh! The pleasant noise of the victory!" Wise Bitter-Gourd smiled on the grounds where he had fallen down, as he experienced peace after lot many days.

"I don't understand how is the digestion working, when whole body is shut down?" Chubby Cauliflower asked as he stood up from the place he fell down.

"She is unconscious not dead." Lemon spoke sarcastically, stating the obvious.

The other cars following them behind them came to a halt and few vegetable soldiers descended from it. They were surprised to see it was their protectors who were travelling in their front vehicle. They had expected to be those traitor bread loafs who were busy circling their small intestine for an opportunity to attack it again.

Even the protectors were pleasantly surprised to see it was their soldiers who were following them and not some bread loafs.

"Are you patrolling?" Wise Bitter-Gourd stood up and asked as he saw the soldiers approaching them.

"We are sir. Indeed!" The soldier spoke as he saluted the protectors, "Loafs tried to attack the intestine once in your absence. We defeated them badly. We crushed them. We started patrolling after that. We have random sighting of loafs when it's usually day and when it's usually night time."

That was a big shock for the protectors. They thought everybody would be tied up in the Toilet jail.

"Everything is fine in intestine?" Lemon asked shocked.

"Everything is perfect in intestine and everybody is safe."

"And my son?" Lady Finger asked hurriedly.

"Your son is currently sleeping peacefully, mam." one of the soldier addressed Mrs Lady Finger.

Mrs Lady Finger clenched her heart over-whelmed on hearing that. "That's wonderful news to my ears."

"Nobody's in the Toilet jail then?" Lemon asked surprised still not believing a word.

"Only the breads who attacked us." The soldier said in a clear voice and with a straight face.

"That means those brown and white breads were just tom-telling us a false story." Nerdy Spinach Leaf spoke as he started to realise the truth.

"But why?" Mrs Lady Finger asked confused, but relieved never-the-less

"So that we would surrender ourselves to them without a fight. Then they would use us as an exchange for small intestine with soldiers." Bitter Gourd concluded. Breads were not that dumb after all!

"That makes sense!" they all smiled as they walked towards their home after the crazy journey.

****

Discreet is all Apple was hoping, it would be. Lantern in his hand burning bright like an orange dot in all the blackness. There were seas of tent lying on the opposite side of the river in front of his eyes. He could just cross the bridge and set all tents with the fire in lantern.

That would also be an excellent revenge for his son's death. Breads were dumb and lazy. They wouldn't even get to know till it would be too late. Still he wasn't dumb enough to try.

He had send Banana to the backyard to bring their small boat parked in garage. Wonder what was taking him so long? Little did he know Banana was engrossed in enjoying himself to the treat of watching Mrs. Lady Finger balancing herself on wooden plank with three jugs like a ballerina. He was blown away. Strawberry or his ex-beetroot were too darlings to be able do that. It was weird though seeing his ex-Beetroot all transformed in blood, swirling in circles in the jug. After the show had ended and Mrs. Lady Finger had climbed down, he took the boat and rushed back in front. Apple gave him a strange look and snatched the boat from his hand.

Apple junior was bossy. Though apple senior was just idiot, apple junior was bossy and idiot. Both father and son duo was unbearable, and now that his son had died, his desire for revenge had made him gone crazy.

They all, all would imply all the fruit protectors except the strawberry and bunch of grapes walked towards the edge of the river. The bunch of Grapes would have joined them too. But she was too sleepy. Like mothers-like daughters. They all loved to sleep. Strawberry on other hand was too delicate for such adventure.

Apple junior lowered the boat in the river, and orange hopped in it followed by others. Cranberry, not missing a single beat to show how ferocious she was, jumped right from a stone into the boat. She shook the entire boat and everybody lost their footing. Apple looked at her bitterly, "That was discreet much? You are going to wake their entire army."

Cranberry ignored him and took her seat in the boat.

Everybody took to rowing the boat towards the opposite side of river where all the tents lay. They were fast approaching those seas of tents, sprawled out rows after rows in a huge stretch as far as their sight could go. Their lazy enemies lay inside that tent.

There was only one lantern amongst them, which the apple held. Too many lanterns wouldn't be discreet much. From a distance they would look like flickering red dots. They docked the boat on the other side. They tried their best not to make the noise below their feet by stepping on the dead skin cells. Apples and other protectors cautiously jumped from one bush to another and hid behind it. Apple looked over the bush to make sure they were in clear. The leftover breads were busy snoring in tents too tired from their travel.

"How were these lazy people even going to compete with us? You have been unnecessarily worrying?" Cranberry uttered to the Apple.

"By their sheer overwhelming number of size and weight. They are still twenty to one of us. In spite of half of them leaving. They can just sit on us and squeeze us alive. They are so huge." Apple junior murmured back.

"Plus I have heard they have earthworms and loads of other germs to rot us. Breads don't need themselves to do dirty work. They have these earthworms to infest us."

"Yes 270 types." Orange said in her orangy voice.

"You have been spending too much time with that Nerdy Spinach Leaf, haven't you?" Apple junior asked her acidly.

"Yeah! He is cute!" Orange blushed, a dark orange tone.

"Focus." Apple junior called her off acidly.

"You forgot leeches." Cranberry fuelled further.

"Oh yes! Those leeches!" Orange scrunched up her face in disgust.

"They must be taking away your beauty." Cranberry sniggered, "You act all girly like strawberry when you are with that leaf."

Orange scowled not appreciating her humour.

The tents reeked of luxury. They were extremely huge. It was more of glamping then camping. They hiked towards the last tent at the back. Apple knew that the earthworms were in the far-off rows, because considering how noisy they are; hardly any buzzing or hissing noises could be heard in their house. Standing outside each tent at the back, they tried to hear buzzing noise if any coming out from insides of the tent, they were highly disappointed. None of the back tents held any worms which was weird. If none of the tents had worms then where were those clusters of hideous worms hidden? They huffed in disappointment and Apple decided to put the tents on fire with just breads in it.

"I hate doing this but I have to", he told everyone before lowering his lantern and setting the ropes of tent on fire. Pretty soon whole tent was engulfed in fire. They could hear screeches and howling of breads from insides. They could vividly see the breads being toasted, turning black and ashes falling on ground.

After setting two tents on fire, Apple went on to burn many others to a crisp.

"Gross! I cannot believe we killed someone!" Cranberry muttered sourly.

"My conscious is pricking me." Orange squeaked.

Fire doused off. Screeches and screaming of breads halted and they could see half toasted and burnt breads on the ground.

The Bread in the tents ahead of now burnt tents stirred in their sleep. Their sleep was being disturbed.

They squirmed in their dreams. They believed they saw a few flames of yellow fire with his half closed- half opened eyes. Even the heat had become unbearable. He knew there was a heavy drought in the body, but this was intense and too sudden! Where were all his lower ranked bread soldiers to fan him now? They were always running behind and ahead of him to fan him. But where were those Half-baked pieces of loafs now? He snarled under his breath. But then he went back to his dream; of being covered up with a thick layer of butter. His roommate too fluttered opened his eyes as smoke hit his nostrils. He thought it might be…well he didn't think too much and went back to sleep.

The three breads in the tent besides that tent, though were curious to know, why suddenly there was so much smoke, they refused to move. The three breads had decided internally that; no matter what happens; they won't leave the tent, in fear, that they would receive some more work. And they did not desire that at all. Same was the case with tents ahead of them. The breads in those tents ahead could hear faint noises and smell faint smoke.

"Do you smell a smoke?" A loaf asked his fellow loaf.

"No! I don't", fellow loaf back answered sleepily.

"Not even faintly?" he asked curiously.

"No, I think you are dreaming of having nightmare of being roasted in barbeque again."

*****

In the tent besides theirs, "Do you smell a faint smoke?" A loaf asked another,

"Yes indeed." The other loaf answered back sincerely.

"Can you go and check it?"

"Yes indeed." He picked up his lantern and went outside to check but he didn't see anything so he came back and went to sleep.

Meanwhile the fruits rushed for cover behind bushes when the bread soldier came out of his tent. Thankfully the fire and smoke from the back tents had doused off till then.

But while running, Orange was taking a lot of time to roll and keep up with the Apple. So Apple just kicked it hard and it rolled ferociously. Orange rolled and rolled deeper and ahead of where he was supposed to stop. It rolled beyond the bushes they were hiding in. It rolled much deeper in the woods.

She fell in a pit. She rolled in a pit of faces."Ew!" She exclaimed "Brown goo' is hanging from my orange skin?" she huffed in disgust. "Nasty stuff." She pouted. She was stomping and wailing now.

Apple looked apprehensive. She was attracting attention, 'Shsh! Keep it down." He whispered to her.

"But there is brown goo hanging from my orange skin," She howled.

Apple was so scared orange would expose them, but thankfully nobody noticed.

Orange looked above where she was standing. She was standing below a wooden cabinet. Something striked her and she screamed happily.

"OMG! Is this 'we hit the jackpot' moment? Jackpot!" She bounced and screamed happily.

Apple glared at now dancing Orange frustratingly. "What was wrong with her?" he wondered

"Is this jackpot? I think it is!" She was now singing and swinging her waist and hips erratically to it. "She has gone bonkers!" Apple face-palmed himself frustratingly.

"Or has she?" Cranberry asked creepily, staring at a wooden cabin below which the orange was bouncing.

"Hear carefully." Creepy cranberry said, "You will hear the earthworms buzzing from that house!" She said, pointing towards the bamboo house.

Apple looked where Cranberry was looking, and a shock of delight tingled in his body. It was indeed a jackpot. It was well-hidden cabinet behind tall the shrubs and the bushes, quite invisible from all the other angles. It was impossible to notice if not looked properly. It would be visible only to sharp eyes.

Orange rolled out of the pit full of brown goo.

Apple walked few paces and stood in front of the wooden house. He looked at others with evil glint in his eyes. Hissing and buzzing noises of earthworms were clearly coming from the house.

"All right guys! Let's do it. Let's kill those worms!"

Orange bounced up the stairs. Others except Apple junior climbed up too and reached the porch of wooden house. The hissing noises dynamically increased. Orange looked inside from the glass window and saw clusters and clusters of worms wiggling and jiggling in their individual sheds. Each shed was occupied by clusters of 3-4 worms wiggling and jiggling in their places. Apple who was standing down whispered quietly in air, "I recommend you guys to come down quickly. I am setting this place on fire." While others climbed down, Orange rolled down. Apple ignited the supporting pillar on which wooden house was erected with his torch. The wood caught the flame and soon the whole hut was on fire. Literally! Flares fluttered and blazed.

"Good job lads. Great destruction. Now let's head back before those lazy people wake up."

****

Chapter 19

Colour of Juices!!!!!!!!

The time when it's usually dawn, a huge earthworm was crawling towards where junior Apple was sprawled across the sofa of their living room. Besides him was Apple the senior. Other protectors too had dozed off in their respective bed after all night's activities.

Slowly and steadily the whole house was getting infested with different types of worms.

A screech from other room woke up both the apples with a start. The Orange was bouncing, either trying to sit on a worm or was trying to get away from it.

Whereas both the Apples tried to jump from the couch when they saw a large earthworm right in front of their face, with its mouth wide open, ready to take a juicy bite of them.

A kitchen knife landed on their window with a thump. The whole house was now infested with worms. A chaos erupted. Everyone came rushing from their rooms and were running here and there, some jumping on chairs.

Cranberry went to kitchen and gathered all the knives in kitchen and passed it to others. Strawberry and banana gathered kids and hid them under the coffee tables and couches and beds to escape the knives scooping in now through broken windows. But soon the kids saw the earthworms crawling towards them under all the tables and couches, which made them jump out from those places.

"So breads finally woke up," Apple wondered as he tried to kill the earthworms with the kitchen knives, which were busy scooping towards their house from the air, creating cracks in walls and woods when they landed in them. Attack from opponents was a full-fledged one. Kitchen Knives to earthworms flying in air or crawling in their lawns, Bread's attack was everywhere in their abode.

Earthworms hanging on sticks and pointed knives were scooping in like cats and dogs. From a distance loud noise of Calcium Swords falling heavy on stone could be heard.

"The enemies are busy breaking our stone wall!" Tomatoes hollered.

"Gather the army!" Apple junior barked the orders.

"Our army have already aligned outside the house." Tomato hollered back and left the mansion.

"O' good lord! Save our house!" Raspberry wept with tears in her eyes.

'Save yourself first, doofus!' Cranberry said annoyed as she attacked another earthworm with one of knives they had in their kitchen.

Apples along with orange went down in their basement of the house to carry crates of supplies for war upstairs at the murder hole on the terrace of third floor.

'It's war time mates, and best way to destroy bread is to infect them with fungus. It is like a bread poison."

Apple and Orange carried the fungus crates to the terrace where army had stationed themselves under directions of tomato. While few soldiers had stationed themselves in front of murder hole carved in wall, others took the terrace wide open. Apples and Oranges kept their crates down and opened them and distributed the inside stuff amongst the army.

The bread army were busy hitting their stone wall with their calcium sword. Tomato had stationed few soldiers downstairs too behind the wall as first line of defence. They all were carrying their calcium and iron swords along with shredders and mixers to churn the breads to crumbs. Soldiers of Both sides were wearing silver protective armours.

Tomato was doing a great job as a commanding officer. "On my command!" Tomato bellowed. The soldiers straightened their backs alert.

"Dip." Tomato commanded. The soldiers dipped their calcium arrows in fungus, and then they lighted the arrow on fire with a lantern.

"Ready?" Tomato barked. All soldiers nodded.

"Nock." Tomato barked the orders. All the soldiers placed the burning arrows in the string.

"Mark." All the soldiers now pointed the arrows towards the breads they wanted to toast.

"Draw." Now all soldiers pulled the stretching strings of arrow.

"Loose." All arrows went flying towards their marked enemies who had managed to now successfully take down most of the wall. They burned and yelped in pain. Smoke started evaporating from their bodies. First they turned golden brown and then they turned crisp black in a blink of eyes. Their ashes fell in a heap on the ground.

"Nock-Mark-Draw-Loose." The soldiers re-did the entire process again as commanded by Tomato after having dipped the arrow in fungus. Many of the breads collapsed in heaps of black ash after turning in golden brown again. They had to do this fast since once bread manages to break down the wall they would ripe open all the fruits with their mixers and juicers. They had already taken half the stone wall down.

"Oh yes baby! That's how it's done!" Banana clapped, cheered and fist pumped the air.

But sadly their attack was short lived as almost the entire stone wall was now broken and the remaining breads were ushering in towards the soldiers of first line of defence.

"Close the gates." Banana commanded.

"We don't have a gate, you idiot!" Apple senior scolded, looking at him severely.

"Oh yeah! Sorry about that." Banana bit back his tongue.

Both the armies ran towards each other with their weapons like shredder, juicer and mixer ready in their hands for attack. They both jumped at each other and now were just breathing down each other's neck. They both were attacking each other mercilessly. It was an unfriendly sight. It was impossible to know who took the lead from upstairs and who were at first. Though their army were successful in shredding few Bread soldiers to crumbs.

"Yes!" All the protestors shouted from upstairs and clapped. But sadly breads were not the ones to take any defeat lying down; they were equally capable of giving a tough fight. They were juicing fruits left, right and centre by their juicer machines. They were randomly opening on them their latest mixers and juicers. They sliced open few fruits with knives. They also let loose many earthworms on them. Many fruits were bitten by those earthworms. Those fruits died on the spot.

Now the soldiers on terrace standing in front of the murder hole unloaded rocks coated with boiling oil on the breads to fry them. When the rock dipped in boiling oil touched the breads they stirred and burned under it until smoke started coming out of their body and they turned crispy golden brown and finally falling into a black heap on the ground.

Every protector clapped on seeing the black ash. The soldiers in front of the murder hole loaded another boiling rock from it and then some more. Many bread soldiers melted on ground, smoke evaporating from their bodies.

But suddenly Bread soldiers were outnumbering fruits soldiers and that was a matter of concern. All their efforts seemed fruitless. All the fruits were falling down with juices flowing out of their body. There was maroon of raspberry soldiers mixing with orange of orange soldiers. The pink of strawberry's had created a puddle which mixed with reds of tomatoes. The cranberries were putting up a great fight but even their dark red colour was dripping everywhere. Even bananas were mashed down with shredders and Apples sliced open. Still they were fighting bravely. It was a dark sight.

While Strawberry protector had tears in her eyes, Raspberry protector could not take it anymore and puked in the nearby plotted plant on seeing her army cut open so brutally. Fruits had lost the battle. Most of their armies were destroyed. Remaining were not enough. Breads number were still hundreds while they were just handful.

All protectors looked at each other with a heart-broken face. It was time to surrender and end the war. But before they could make a move towards surrendering, breads started melting. They faded slowly without any assistance. Ditto with worms! Their enemy precisely just vanished in thin air to their surprise.

The heat in the air decreased, and there was a soothing rainfall all over the liver.

People used to always stare at Tee. Where ever she looked people had their eyes on her. Earlier she thought people used to stare her because she was special. After all, they never stared anybody else, just her. But slowly she started gaining weight. Still people stared her wherever she went. She was convinced now they were staring her because she suddenly gained weight. She felt ugly. She didn't feel special at all. After all they only stared her and not others. But one fine day something daunted on her. She held her face embarrassment on the sudden realisation. How could she have never realised that before? People only stared at her because primarily she was the one who used to start staring at them first; she unconsciously or probably unintentionally was trying to figure out what they were thinking. Like staring them would give her their perception. She was always a people pleaser. They merely just stared back. That was so embarrassing!

Today also people were giving her weird stares. But today she was convinced, nobody stared her because she stared them first, because, she had kept her head down, the whole day, refusing to look up. What started out as discreet weird stare broke out in full gawking as the day progressed, and at the end of school time everybody gave her disgusting stares. Like right now nobody stood beside her at the bus-stop. They all kept a safe distance from her. They had seen her full-fledged digging her nose. Also there were rumours of lemons and Cauliflower coming out of her nose and ears. Maybe these were side-effects of some voodoo gone wrong, they thought. Or there was something really wrong in her body. Anyways she was a freak! Some dismissed all those rumours, being the good people, that they were, who refused to indulge in such gossips.

Her friends pitied her from a distance. They looked at each other awkwardly, took a gulp and walked towards her. They were committing social suicide by walking towards her, but clearly their friend looked like she was about to cry. And they weren't that horrible people who would just ignore their friend in need. They were friends indeed!

They obviously dismissed the rumours of lemon coming out of her nose and ears. Others, who had seen it, described it very animatedly. But they knew better, that they were just bunch of attention seeker. Also they knew their friend better. She would never do any sort of voodoo stuff. That they were certain of! Yes she shouldn't have taken so many pills unsupervised. She didn't even follow the instructions at back of the bottle. She was evidently overdosing on them. But they could understand her. She wanted to get slim. She wanted to look pretty like them, and staying hungry all the time was difficult. It took them months to master that art after all.

Tee saw her friends walking towards her when suddenly blue, red and white dots started dancing in front of her eyes. Her head started spinning. Her vision became weak. Now black spots started dancing in front of her eyes. She blacked out and fell down on the bus stop. Her friends witnessed their friend falling on the ground. They rushed and ran towards her.

Teachers and principal rushed outside. Thankfully her breath was still going on. They took her indoors and placed her on the couch, while one of her teacher started rubbing her feet. Her friends fanned her. Some of them threw water on her face. But to no use. Her ears and nose were bright red while her eyes were fast shut. The Principal hastily called her parents as well as an ambulance.

"It might have happened because of these." J confessed guiltily, as she fished out the pills bottle from the tee's bag.

"These are hunger suppressant pills." The teacher said examining the bottle upside down. "You should have reported the authorities."

Her friends cast their heads down in shame.

Sirens of ambulance could be heard from a distance before it halted in front of the school gates. Tee was adjusted in a stretcher before she was taken to a hospital in that ambulance.

Her parents arrived in the hospital shortly. After inquiring at the reception, they dashed straight towards the examination room in the hospital where Tee was kept under observation.

Her mum felt incredibly guilty and continuously fumbled with her hands. She knew Tee was disturbed with her weight and must have done something drastic. She could have avoided it, by giving Tee proper counselling. Her husband immediately rushed from work after hearing the disturbing news. They waited for doctor to exit the examination room and address them.

The principal walked up to them and showed them the bottle, "Did you know about these pills?" She asked them kindly as they were visibly distressed. A shadow of fright passed on mum's face. She had no idea about the pills. Even his dad shook his head in denial.

"These are hunger suppressant pills. Apparently Tee was overdosing on them." Principal spoke slowly. Both the parent looked at each other confused.

While her father clenched his jaw in terror, her mum would break in tears at any moment. The principal tried to pacify the disturbed couple.

A grim-faced doctor in a lab coat exited the room and walked up-to the couple with a notepad in his hand.

“Are you Tee’s parents?” he asked soberly while both of them nodded.

“Do not worry, she is fine.” He consoled them. “But I am afraid we will have to keep her in observation due to some unnatural activities happening in her liver. It was quite peculiar to be honest and it completely confused me. There are extreme amount of bread particles in her liver. There is lot of heat in the organ itself and extreme dehydration. Also we found from our x-rays and other examination test, that her liver organ is infested with earthworms.

All the three adults standing beside each other in front of the doctor looked shocked as they soaked in all the information. “Also we found lots of hunger suppressant pills in her stomach. She had been starving herself and hence her blood level went down,” the doctor continued. “Her sugar went down, her heart slowed down and eventually her blood level fell down.”

Mum clenched her fist in apprehension. Her face contorted in anguish. She could even feel her husband’s anxiety from besides.

“But do not worry we have sucked out all the bread from the body and hydrated the entire liver. We have also sterilised all the worms from her body. We also infused blood in Tee’s body by keeping her on blood bottles. Now her body will heal better.”

Hearing that was like waves gushing on dry lands. Tee’s parents heaved a sigh of relief. She would be better. Well eventually though!

The doctor moved towards other patients then but not before adding, “Also her nose and ears are quite red and sore,” before moving away.

Few days went by in small intestine. A soldier brought few visitors with him, few vegetables who would go on to become their new protectors to be precise.

On seeing them, the existing protectors welcomed them. They also took a hint to start packing their bags for it was time for them to sacrifice themselves.

Mrs Lady Finger kissed his son goodbye. He was comfortable and cheerful with his new family of soldiers and didn’t cry for his mum.

He was at home with them. They took care of him and played with him.

Most importantly he was safe and sound with them. The whole intestine was!"

It was times for six of them to sacrifice themselves in digestion and make place for the new vegetables.

By taking oaths Lemon, Broccoli and the Bean family consisting of kidney bean, soya bean and green beans, took the throne. After coronation ceremony and feasting whole night, as soon as dawn broke and first sight of light broke the skin and entered the body, the six vegetables walked towards the digestion.

****

www.ingramcontent.com/pod-product-compliance
Ingram Content Group UK Ltd.
Pitfield, Milton Keynes, MK11 3LW, UK
UKHW040038200726
13845UKWH00054B/487

9 789387 131439